PUBLIC HEALTH IN THE 21ST CENTURY

PNEUMONIA

SYMPTOMS, DIAGNOSIS AND TREATMENT

PUBLIC HEALTH IN THE 21ST CENTURY

Additional books in this series can be found on Nova's website
under the Series tab.

Additional E-books in this series can be found on Nova's website
under the E-books tab.

PUBLIC HEALTH IN THE 21ST CENTURY

PNEUMONIA

SYMPTOMS, DIAGNOSIS AND TREATMENT

MICAELA L. SUÁREZ
AND
STEFFANI M. ORTEGA
EDITORS

Nova Science Publishers, Inc.
New York

For permission to use material from this book please contact us:
Telephone 631-231-7269; Fax 631-231-8175
Web Site: http://www.novapublishers.com

Library of Congress Cataloging-in-Publication Data

Pneumonia : symptoms, diagnosis, and treatment / editors, Micaela L. Suarez
and Steffani M. Ortega.
p. ; cm.
Includes bibliographical references and index.
ISBN 978-1-61209-685-8 (hardcover : alk. paper)
1. Pneumonia. I. Suarez, Micaela L. II. Ortega, Steffani M.
[DNLM: 1. Pneumonia. WC 202]
RC771.P686 2011
616.2'41--dc22

2011004271

Published by Nova Science Publishers, Inc. †New York

Contents

Preface

Pneumonia, an inflammatory condition of the lung, is one of the most common serious infections, causing two million deaths annually among young and old alike. This new book studies the symptoms, diagnoses and treatment of pneumonia. Topics discussed include the modes of supportive treatment in patients with pneumonia; pneumocystis jirovecii in AIDS patients; nosocomial pneumonia surveillance and prevention in PICU and NICU; ventilator-associated pneumonia; community acquired staphylococcal pneumonia associated with influenza and radiological patterns of pulmonary infections.

Chapter I – *Pneumocystis jirovecii* (formerly *Pneumocystis carinii* sp. f. *hominis*) is an unusual fungus exhibiting pulmonary tropism and a highly defined host specificity. It is generally regarded as an opportunistic microorganism causing severe and often fatal pneumonia in AIDS patients. However, with the currently rising number of patients receiving immunosuppressive therapies for malignancies, allogeneic organ transplantations and autoimmune diseases, *Pneumocystis* pneumonia is becoming more and more recognized in non-HIV immunosuppressed individuals. The clinical presentation in HIV-infected patients may differ from that in other immunocompromised patients and its diagnosis continues to be challenging because no combination of symptoms, signs, blood chemistries, or radiographic findings is specific of *Pneumocystis* pneumonia. In addition, as *P. jirovecii* cannot be grown in culture from clinical specimens, the diagnosis of *Pneumocystis* pneumonia continues to rely on the microscopic demonstration of the characteristic organisms using conventional cytochemical or immunofluorescence staining in respiratory samples. These methods are useful when the organism burden is relatively high but they are insufficient for reliable detection when there is a small parasite load. Therefore, in an attempt to improve diagnosis of *Pneumocystis* pneumonia, more sensitive molecular techniques such as conventional and quantitative PCR have been developed. Using molecular technique mutations in both the gene encoding dihydropteroate synthetase, the target enzyme of sulfonamides, and the gene encoding cytochrome B, conferring potential atovaquone resistance, have been demonstrated. However, their clinical relevance on treatment failure has not yet been determined. Co-trimoxazole, an association of trimethoprim and sulfamethoxazole, pentamidine isethionate or atovaquone has been extensively prescribed for the prophylaxis and therapy of *Pneumocystis* pneumonia.

Nevertheless, co-trimoxazole is currently regarded as the drug of choice for prophylaxis and therapy of any form or severity of *Pneumocystis* pneumonia. Looming on the horizon is the specter of resistance to co-trimoxazole and atovaquone, but there are few options for other alternative treatments. A prompt appropriate therapy is probably the most crucial factor in improving the prognosis of this devastating pneumonia for which care providers must continue to maintain a high index of suspicion in immunocompromised patients at risk. The management of *Pneumocystis* pneumonia remains a major challenge for all physicians caring for immunosuppressed patients.

Chapter II – Pneumonia is one of the most common serious infections, causing two million deaths annually among young children in low-income countries. It is the largest killer, accounting for 28 to 34% of all child deaths below five years of age in low income countries and is an important cause of mortality in the elderly in high-income countries. Despite availability of effective antibiotic treatment the mortality remains 6 to 12% in patients admitted to hospital with community acquired pneumonia and over 50% in patients admitted to the intensive care unit (figures from the United Kingdom). The objective of this review is to summarize evidence for the effectiveness of modes of supportive treatment in patients with pneumonia. Supportive treatment explored in patients with pneumonia includes oxygen in a variety of applications, fluid therapy regimens, chest physiotherapy, steroid treatment, granulocyte colony stimulating factor treatment, surfactant application and vitamins A, C and D, zinc, protein and calorie supplements. Studies showed that management of patients with monitoring of oxygen levels and oxygen delivery guided by oxygen saturation levels can reduce hospitalisation. In children four randomised controlled trials compared oxygen delivery methods and found that nasal prongs and nasopharyngeal catheters were found to be similar in effectiveness and safety. Review of trials, which assessed the accuracy of clinical signs indicating hypoxemia found that no single clinical sign or symptom accurately identified hypoxemia. Vitamin C supplementation in critically ill patients was associated with lower mortality and reduced respiratory symptom score in one trial. Steroid application was associated with reduction of mortality and need for mechanical ventilation in people with pneumocystis jiroveci pneumonia but there has been insufficient evidence supporting their use in other forms of pneumonia. Use of granulocyte colony stimulating factor application was not associated with reduction of mortality in a meta-analysis of 6 studies. Six trials investigating vitamin A showed no significant reduction in mortality or duration of hospital stay but demonstrated a 39% reduction in antibiotic first line failure (OR 0.65: 95% CI 0.42 to 1.01). Trials using supplementation with zinc did not show consistent benefit. For fluid regimes, chest physiotherapy, vitamin D and protein and calorie supplements there has been a lack of evidence for an influence on outcome and further research is required.

Chapter III – Ventilator associated pneumonia (VAP), the second most common hospital-acquired infection among pediatric and neonatal intensive care unit (PICU and NICU) patients, is defined as the pneumonia that develops later than or at 48 hours after the patient has been placed on mechanical ventilation. In spite of the fact that its incidence is higher in adult patient's intensive care unit, VAP is associated with increased morbidity, length of PICU and NICU stay, antibiotic use and costs also in pediatric population. The lack of a gold standard for the diagnosis of VAP makes an interpretation of the literature complex, and differences in the incidence of VAP occur as a result of the definitions used and people doing the surveillance. As in other hospitals, in our experience the incidence of VAP seemed increase after the implementation of a VAP surveillance program. We have measured in terms of quality the impact of a specific program of prevention and surveillance of VAP in pediatric population, in a patient-centred model of healthcare assistance. Since 2000 to 2004 VAP represented the 8.66% of all hospital-acquired infections in our PICU. Gram-negative bacilli represented the most of isolates (*Escherichia coli and Pseudomonas aeruginosa*). The medium values of our PICU indexes were 5.52 for the Physiologic Stability Index (PSI), 5.9 for the Pediatric Risk of Mortality Score (PRISM) and 13 (class II) for the Therapeutic Intervention Scoring System (TISS). In NICU data we found 7.50 VAP per thousand days of mechanical ventilation, with very-low-birth-weight infants suffering the highest incidence rate. The nosocomial infection preventive measures, principally the hand hygiene of the health-care personnel and visitors, the correct asepsis before invasive procedures, the adequacy of antibiotics policy, and the correct nutrition of our children have demonstrated to reduce the risk of suffering a hospital-acquired infection even in 50%.

Chapter IV – Ventilator-associated pneumonia (VAP) is the most frequent intensive care unit (ICU)-acquired infection, occurring in 6 to 52% of patients intubated for more than 48 hours. It is associated with high mortality and morbidity, prolonged lengths of hospitalisation, and also increased cost of health-care. Because of the huge disease burden and the resultant attributable morbidity and mortality, so much importance is given for accurate diagnosis and treatment of this condition. In the critically ill patients on mechanical ventilation, the clinical signs and symptoms of pneumonia are non-specific and varied. Consequently, the diagnosis is difficult and most often delayed. The lack of a "gold standard" for diagnosis further compounds this problem. Although many clinical, radiological, microbiological and histopathological criteria have been suggested by various workers, all of them have certain inherent demerits. The management of patients with VAP is so challenging because of the increased association of multi-drug resistant organisms with this condition. Several treatment strategies and guidelines have been recommended by expert panels for appropriate treatment of these patients without contributing to development of drug resistance. Significant advances have been made in this field over the past few decades, which will reviewed in this chapter to improve our understanding of the symptoms of VAP and help us to accurately diagnosis and treat this condition.

Chapter V– Bacterial pneumonia complicating influenza has been recognized at least since the 19th century. In this setting *Staphylococcus aureus* is one of the most common offenders and is associated with a potentially severe disease accompanied by high rates of morbidity and mortality. The recent increase in staphylococcal infections caused by community-acquired methicillin-resistant *Staphylococcus aureus* (CA-MRSA), has been increasingly recognized to be associated with community associated pneumonia (CAP). This type of pneumonia affects mainly a younger age group, frequently follows infection with influenza, and is often severe, requiring hospitalization and causing death in a significant proportion of those affected. Recognizing the role of *Staphylococcus aureus* in general and CA-MRSA in particular as important causes of pneumonia after influenza infection may decrease the delay before the institution of appropriate antimicrobial therapy, which in turn should contribute to improved outcome of this severe disease. This article reviews the epidemiology, clinical features, diagnosis, and therapies for staphylococcal pneumonia complicating influenza virus infection.

Staphylococcus aureus (SA) is a relatively uncommon cause of community acquired pneumonia thought to account for only 3–5% of cases [1, 2]. *S. aureus* pneumonia is, however, a well-recognized complication occurring after infection with influenza both following seasonal and pandemic types and other viral pneumonia (varicella, adeno-virus) in children and young adults. *S. aureus* pneumonia complicating influenza has accounted for a large number of deaths [3–6]. Morens et al. reviewed bacterial culture results from 96 autopsy series, from civil and military sources from the 1918-1919 influenza pandemic, a total of 5266 positive culture results- were found. *S.* aureus was the third most common bacterial pathogen identified, accounting for 8.1% of deaths occurring in these series [7]. Recent data is emerging to suggest an increase in the frequency of SA pneumonia. Possibly the first documented cases in North America were reported by Francis et. al[8]. All 4 patients in that small case series had a syndrome characterized by an influenza or influenza-like prodrome, shock and cavitary lesion. One of the patients succumbed to the infections while the others recovered after a prolonged hospital course Finelli et al.[9] reported 166 influenza- associated pediatric deaths in the years 2004-2007 pointing to the seriousness of this super-infection. Reports of bacterial co-infection of influenza increased from 6% in 2004–2005, to 15% in 2005-2006 and to 34% in 2006–2007. *S aureus* was isolated from a sterile site or from the endotracheal tube in 1 case in 2004–2005, from 3 cases in 2005–2006, and from 22 cases in 2006–2007. Another trend observed in this study was the significant role of methicillin-resistant *S aureus* (MRSA) accounting for 64% of SA isolates, with the majority of cases occurring in the latest reporting period [9]. A survey of 59 US hospitals involving 4543 patients with culture-positive pneumonia between January 2002 and January 2004 [10] identified MRSA as a potential pathogen in CAP (8.9%). Moreover, *Staphylococcus aureus* was the only pathogen identified to be independently associated with mortality according to a logistic regression analysis in this study. Kallen et al. [11] reported a survey conducted by The Infectious Diseases Society of America's Emerging Infections Network (EIN) in 2007, revealing episodes of severe *S. aureus* community acquired pneumonia (CAP) diagnosed during the 2006-2007 influenza season. CAP was defined as "pneumonia requiring hospitalization of an outpatient not residing in a long-term care facility." Nearly half of the responding surveyed members (509- 47%) reported treating a total of 440 adults and 117 children who were hospitalized because of *S. aureus* CAP. Of these patients, nearly a half (49%) required mechanical ventilation, and 13% succumbed to the infection. In the survey, respondents suspected that a quarter of the patients had an associated influenza infection, on basis of history or clinical findings. However, influenza was confirmed by laboratory testing in only 6% of cases. This report too points to the increased frequency and severity of S A pneumonia complicating viral pneumonia.

The CDC has documented reports from state and local health departments over the last several influenza seasons describing previously healthy children with a severe *s. aureus* CAP [12]. The increasing role of CA-MRSA and high mortality rates are evident in more recent reports, although it is unclear whether they represent heightened awareness and reporting or a real shift in severity.

The mechanisms by which prior influenza infection predisposes to subsequent SA pneumonia is beyond the scope of this manuscript and may involve changes in epithelial defense and changes in epithelial cell wall leading to increased bacterial adherence, changes in the ability of the innate cells to recognize the pathogen, impaired migration or inability of macrophages and white blood cells to eradicate the invading organism [13-15]. The magnitude of the risk depends on the particular strain of influenza virus and the degree of local epithelial damage and immune dysregulation the viral infection induces as well as on the virulence and antibiotic susceptibility of the ensuing SA strains.

Chapter VI – Pulmonary infections still remain the most common infectious cause of mortality in the world, causing around six million deaths per year in the United States where they are the sixth cause of mortality and an important morbid-mortality source. We are therefore facing a problem enormous magnitude in social, economic and above all, health service areas.

In this chapter the authors will refer to pneumonia as an inflammatory-infectious process, although it is necessary to be aware of the existence of other etiological causes of inflammation in the lung that are not specifically mentioned in this chapter. When the authors find a patient presenting fever, cough, tachypnea, and rales on auscultation a clinical diagnosis of infectious pneumonia should be considered although at the same time we know that there are certain pathologies that can clinically mimic the presence of pneumonia. To guide the clinical diagnosis of pneumonia, establish the optimal treatment based on the etiological diagnosis and make an adequate follow up of these patients various diagnostic tests, both invasive and non-invasive, are available to us. Among the complete diagnostic battery used to the study lung infections the 'Gold Standard' test is currently the conventional chest radiograph (CXR). In fact, the American Thoracic Society recommends the practice of a CXR, including posterior/anterior and lateral projectionsfor an adult with suspected pneumonia. So this is the first step that we must take. Just a single study composed of two projections of the patient's chest that will give us valuable information for an initial interpretation. If there is no clinical-radiological correlation or we find complications or abnormal evolution of the infection we can carry out Computed Tomography (CT) or other useful procedures for the management of the pneumonia. Within the range of available non-invasive laboratory tests we should mention sputum and blood culture or serology of infectious agents. On the invasive side we can use transtracheal aspiration, thoracentesis, closed pleural biopsy, bronchoscopy with aspiration and brushing, transbronchial biopsy, percutaneous aspiration and open pulmonary or pleural biopsies.

In: Pneumonia: Symptoms, Diagnosis and Treatment
Editors: M. L. Suarez and S. M. Ortega, pp. 1-36
ISBN: 978-1-61209-685-8

Chapter I

Pneumocystis jirovecii Pneumonia

***Enrique J. Calderón*[1], *José Manuel Varela*[1], *Isabelle Durand-Joly*[2] and *Eduardo Dei-Cas*[2]**
Instituto de Biomedicina de Sevilla and CIBER de Epidemiología y Salud Pública, Internal Medicine Service, Virgen del Rocío University Hospital. Seville, Spain[1]
Parasitology-Mycology Service (EA3609), Biology & Pathology Centre, UDSL, Univ. Lille Nord de France, Lille-2 University Hospital Centre & IFR-142 Institut Pasteur de Lille, France[2]

Abstract

Pneumocystis jirovecii (formerly *Pneumocystis carinii* sp. f. *hominis*) is an unusual fungus exhibiting pulmonary tropism and a highly defined host specificity. It is generally regarded as an opportunistic microorganism causing severe and often fatal pneumonia in AIDS patients. However, with the currently rising number of patients receiving immunosuppressive therapies for malignancies, allogeneic organ transplantations and autoimmune diseases, *Pneumocystis* pneumonia is becoming more and more recognized in non-HIV immunosuppressed individuals. The clinical presentation in HIV-infected patients may differ from that in other immunocompromised patients and its diagnosis continues to be challenging because no combination of symptoms, signs, blood chemistries, or radiographic findings is specific of *Pneumocystis* pneumonia. In addition, as *P. jirovecii* cannot be grown in culture from clinical specimens, the diagnosis of *Pneumocystis* pneumonia continues to rely on the microscopic demonstration of the characteristic organisms using conventional cytochemical or immunofluorescence staining in respiratory samples. These methods are useful when the organism burden is relatively high but they are insufficient for reliable detection when there is a small parasite load. Therefore, in an attempt to improve diagnosis of *Pneumocystis* pneumonia, more sensitive molecular techniques such as conventional and quantitative PCR have been developed. Using molecular technique mutations in both the gene encoding dihydropteroate synthetase, the target enzyme of sulfonamides, and the gene encoding cytochrome B, conferring potential atovaquone resistance, have been demonstrated.

However, their clinical relevance on treatment failure has not yet been determined. Co-trimoxazole, an association of trimethoprim and sulfamethoxazole, pentamidine isethionate or atovaquone has been extensively prescribed for the prophylaxis and therapy of *Pneumocystis* pneumonia.

Nevertheless, co-trimoxazole is currently regarded as the drug of choice for prophylaxis and therapy of any form or severity of *Pneumocystis* pneumonia. Looming on the horizon is the specter of resistance to co-trimoxazole and atovaquone, but there are few options for other alternative treatments. A prompt appropriate therapy is probably the most crucial factor in improving the prognosis of this devastating pneumonia for which care providers must continue to maintain a high index of suspicion in immunocompromised patients at risk. The management of *Pneumocystis* pneumonia remains a major challenge for all physicians caring for immunosuppressed patients.

Introduction and Historical Perspective

Pneumocystis jirovecii, previously known as *Pneumocystis carinii* sp. f. *hominis* [1], is an atypical fungus exhibiting pulmonary tropism and a highly defined host specificity. This microorganism causes opportunistic infection, particularly pneumonia, in patients who have impaired immunity. The general term for clinical disease caused by *Pneumocystis* is pneumocystosis.

Pneumocytsis was originally identified in 1909 by Carlos Chagas in the lungs of guinea pigs that were inoculated with the blood of trypanomiasis patients. Therefore, he erroneously thought that this organism was part of the life cycle of *Trypanosoma cruzi*. One year later, Antonio Carini made a similar description in the lungs of rats infected by *Trypanosoma lewisi*. It was not until 1912 that the Delanoës working at the Pasteur Institute in Paris recognized that *Pneumocystis* in rats represented a unique species and suggested naming the new microorganism *P. carinii* in honor of Antonio Carinii [2].

For seven decades, most investigators thought *Pneumocystis* organisms to be protozoans because they do not look much like fungi base on the histological characteristics of its trophozoite and cyst life forms, fail to grow much in culture, and are not eliminated from patients by treatment with the usual antifungal agents. By contrast, drugs, such as trimethoprim-sulfamethoxazole and pentamidine, which are often useful in treating protozoan infections, are also active against *Pneumocystis*.

Throughout this time *P. carinii* has been regarded as a single protozoan organism capable of infecting a wide variety of animal species [3]. This idea lasted until 1988 when DNA studies were able to identify it as an atypical fungus close to the family of *Aschomycetos* [4]. Subsequent studies using molecular techniques allowed knowing other aspects, as it is a ubiquitous fungus with pulmonary tropism, which colonizes only mammals and that have a high specificity for the host (stenoxenism). In this way, it has been shown in cross-infection experiments that the species of *Pneumocystis* is specific to each type of mammal, with no transmission among mammals of different species [5]. Therefore, human pneumocystosis is not a zoonotic disease, and this notion has important implications for the epidemiology of human-derived *Pneumocystis*. These findings have recently determined the modification of the nomenclature of *Pneumocystis* that colonize and cause infection in humans, formerly known as *P. carinii sp. f. hominis*, and has now been renamed *P. jirovecii* [6], leaving the end of *P. carinii* to the cause of infection in rats.

Pneumocystis is generally regarded as an opportunistic microorganism causing serious pneumonia in immunocompromised patients, especially in those with AIDS. However, *Pneumocystis* was first identified as a human-pathogen in premature or malnourished infants suffering from interstitial plasma cell pneumonia in European countries around World War II, occasionally occurring in epidemics [2,3]. Since then *Pneumocystis* pneumonia (PcP) had only been reported infrequently in individuals with malignancies and solid organ transplantations until the human immunodeficiency virus (HIV) pandemia turned PcP into a major medical and public health problem in the 1980s [2]. During the 1990s, the introduction of highly active antiretroviral therapy (HAART) for HIV infection and *Pneumocystis* chemoprophylaxis reduced the frequency of PcP. Although at the beginning of this century, the incidence of pneumonia caused by this microorganism among subjects with HIV infection has decreased in developed countries, the prevalence of AIDS-related PcP in developing countries remains high and poorly controlled. AIDS-related PcP continues to be a devastating illness among subjects unaware of their HIV infection, persons without access to antiretroviral therapy, among patients who are intolerant or non-adherent, and in occasional cases of failure of prophylaxis [4]. For theses reasons, PcP still remains considered as a principal AIDS-defining illness [7].

Presently, interest in *P. jirovecii* infection goes beyond AIDS patients since with the rising number of patients receiving immunosuppressive therapies for autoimmune diseases, malignancies, allogeneic bone marrow or solid organ transplantations, PcP is more and more recognized in non-HIV immunosuppressed patients [5,6,8]. Underlying conditions associated with PcP in HIV-negative patients include hematologic or solid malignancies, allograft transplantation, autoimmune inflammatory disorders (mainly Wegener granulomatosis and systemic lupus erythematosus), inflammatory bowel disease, protein-calorie malnutrition, and congenital immunodeficiency disorders [5,6,8-12]. Lately, PcP has been reported in patients undergone treatment with new biological tumor necrosis factor-alpha antagonist agents (adalimumab, infliximab, etanercept) and anti-CD20 monoclonal antibody, rituximab [13-16].

However, despite advances in laboratory technology, the diagnosis of PcP continues to be challenging [17]. PcP may be difficult to diagnose owing to nonspecific symptoms and signs, the use of chemoprophylaxis and simultaneous infection with multiple organisms in an immunocompromised individual [18]. On the other hand, few treatment options exist for patients with PcP. Thus, management of PcP remains a major challenge to all physicians caring for these patients.

Life-Cycle

The complete life cycles of any of the species of *Pneumocystis* are not known, but presumably, all resemble the others in the genus. Many investigators have attempted to cultivate *Pneumocystis* using a variety of techniques, but have had limited success, impeding studies of *Pneumocystis*. Pneumonia models in immune-suppressed animals remain the main source of organisms for laboratory studies, yet these approaches have numerous inherent difficulties. Studies of the life cycle of *Pneumocystis* have been based mainly on light and electron microscopic analysis of forms seen in infected lungs or short-term cultures [19] There are two predominant morphologic life cycle forms of *Pneumocystis*, the trophic form

(1-4 μm) and the cystic form (8-10 μm) with three intermediate cyst stages (early, intermediate, and late precysts).

All stages are found in lungs but the trophozoite stage is the vegetative state that predominates over the cystic form during infection by approximately 10:1. During infection, most trophic forms are haploid and it has been hypothesized that trophic forms can conjugate and develop into cysts. The mature cysts contain eight intracystic nuclei (figure 1). It has been suggested that trophic forms originate from the intracystic nuclei of the mature cyst as its ruptures and then undergo vegetative growth or conjugation to re-form the cysts forms. It is further proposed that they may also undergo asexual reproduction through haploid mitosis and binary fission. In an infected host, *Pneumocystis* exists almost exclusively within lung alveoli. The trophic forms attach to the alveolar epithelium trough interdigitation of their membranes. This adherence is characterized by close apposition of the cell surface without fusion of the membranes and strongly promotes proliferation of the organism. *Pneumocystis* maintains an extracellular existence within alveoli, and probably obtains essential nutrients from the alveolar fluid or living cells. The adherence of *Pneumocystis* also inhibits the growth of lung epithelial cells. Although organism attachment to alveoli epithelial cells is essential for *Pneumocystis* infection and propagation, invasion of host cells is uncommon and extrapulmonary pneumocystosis occurs only in the setting of severe immunosuppression.

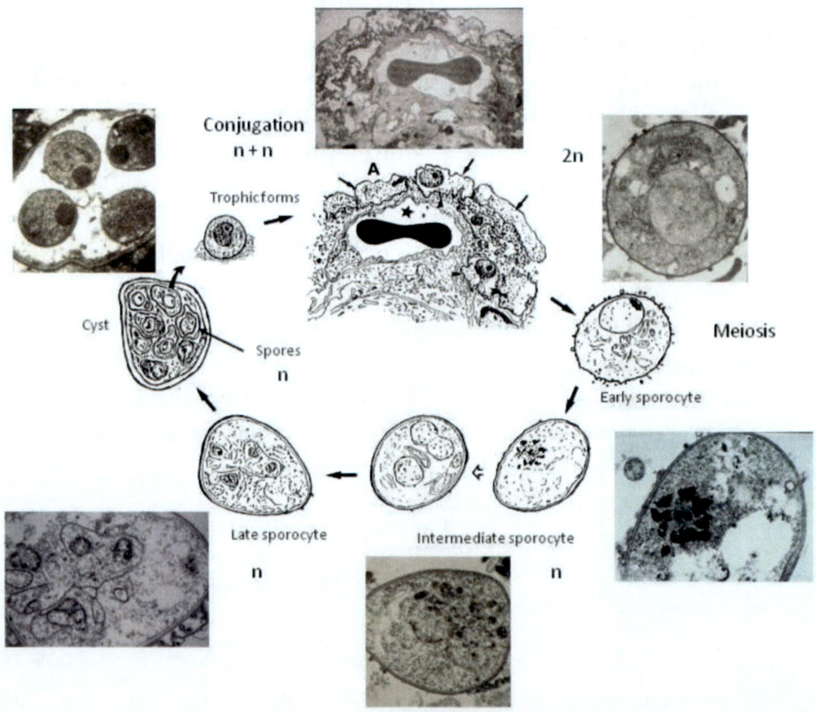

Figure 1. A hypothetical Pneumocystis life cycle illustrated by transmission electron micrographs and corresponding interpretation drawings of organisms developing in mammalian lungs. Mononuclear thin-walled trophic forms (small arrows) are attached to type 1 epithelial alveolar cells. An alveolar capillary vessel was indicated (star). Following conjugation (n+n), trophic forms could evolve into early sporocyte (2n), in which synaptonemal complexes evidenced meiosis. While an electron-lucent layer develops in intermediate sporocytes, mitotic nuclear divisions proceed. An additional mitotic replication leads to a thick-walled late sporocyte containing eight haploid (n) nuclei. In the mature cyst, the eight haploid (n) spores are

fully formed. These forms are able to leave the cyst and subsequently attach to type I alveolar cells. A: alveolar space. (Modified from: Aliouat-Denis et al. Mem Inst Oswaldo Cruz. 2009; 104:419-26. [19]).

Clinical Symptoms and Radiological Findings

Patients with PcP often develop dyspnea, which increases over time; cough productive of clear sputum or nonproductive cough; low grade or no fever; malaise, and sometimes chest tightness or pain. However, the clinical picture in individual patients is variable and many infectious and non-infectious processes can present identically. Also, the general hallmarks of this disease such as fever, shortness of breath, and diffuse infiltrates do not invariably occur, especially early in the course while the disease is mild [18,20,21]. Acute dyspnea with pleuritic chest pain may indicate the development of a pneumothorax, which has been presented in 2% to 4% of patients [22].

In patients infected with HIV, PcP is a common AIDS-defining illness and occurs most frequently in subjects with a CD4+ count less than 200 cells per cubic millimeter. The clinical course is subacute onset with progressive dyspnea, a nonproductive cough, malaise, and low-grade fever. A more acute illness with symptoms including a cough productive with purulent sputum should suggest an alternate infectious diagnosis, such as bacterial pneumonia or tuberculosis.

Non-HIV immunosuppressed patients usually have a more rapid onset than those infected with HIV. PcP usually has a subacute presentation with more insidious involvement in patients with HIV infection than in non-HIV immunosuppressed patients where PcP is much more likely to be an acute illness causing severe respiratory distress that frequently requires mechanical ventilation within the first several days [23,24]. In children, the symptoms of PcP can often be quite subtle, with an increased respiratory rate heralding the first sign of respiratory tract involvement. After a gradual onset, patients present progressive dyspnea, cyanosis, anorexia, weight-loss, and diarrhea whereas cough and fever can be absent [25].

In all cases, a high index of suspicion and a thorough history are key factors in early detection of PcP. Physical examination may reveal tachypnea, tachycardia, and cyanosis. Lung auscultation usually reveals few abnormalities with dry cackles or rhonchi present in less than 50% of patients. Individuals with PcP can be hypoxemic with respiratory alkalosis but can also have normal alveolar-arterial gradients if identified early in the natural history of their disease. Elevated serum levels of lactate dehydrogenase (LDH) have been related with PcP and probably reflects lung parenchymal damage but is not specific. In general, laboratory abnormalities are less severe in HIV-infected patients than in non-HIV immunosuppressed patients [5].

Classic chest radiographic features of PcP, in patients with and without HIV infection, are bilateral, symmetric, fine reticular interstitial infiltrates involving the perihilar areas (figure 2a), becoming more homogenous and diffuse as the severity of the infection increases [18]. However, almost every conceivable radiographic presentation has been linked to PcP, including asymmetrical infiltrates, nodular densities, cavitary lesions, lymphadenopaties, pleural effusions, pneumatoceles, and pneumothorax. Patients who receive aerosolized pentamidine have an increased frequency of upper-lobe infiltrates, pneumothorax, or cystic lesions. Early in the course of PcP, the chest radiograph may be normal in up to 25% of cases [26]. A high-resolution computed tomography scan is more sensitive than a chest radiograph and it may reveal changes suggestive of PcP (figure 2b), as extensive ground-glass attenuation or cystic lesions predominating in perihilar areas, even then chest radiographic findings are normal [27]. While such findings are suggestive, they are not diagnostic. However, a negative high-resolution computed tomography scan may allow exclusion of PcP in such patients.

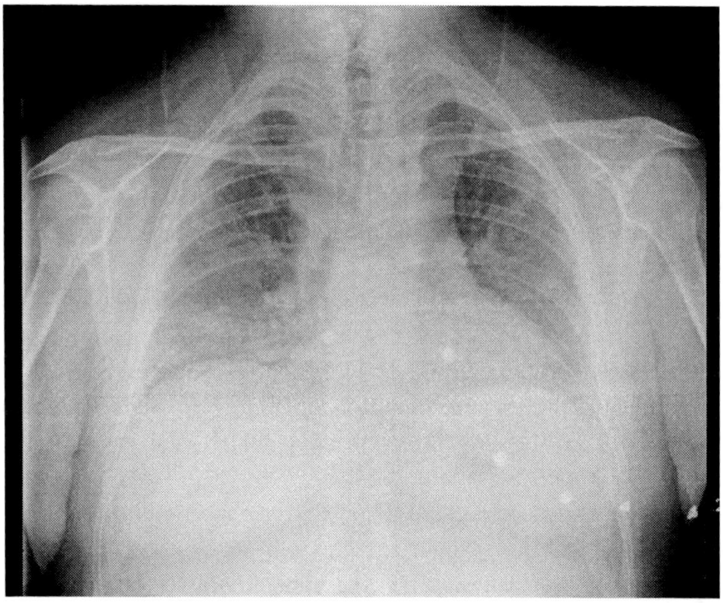

2a

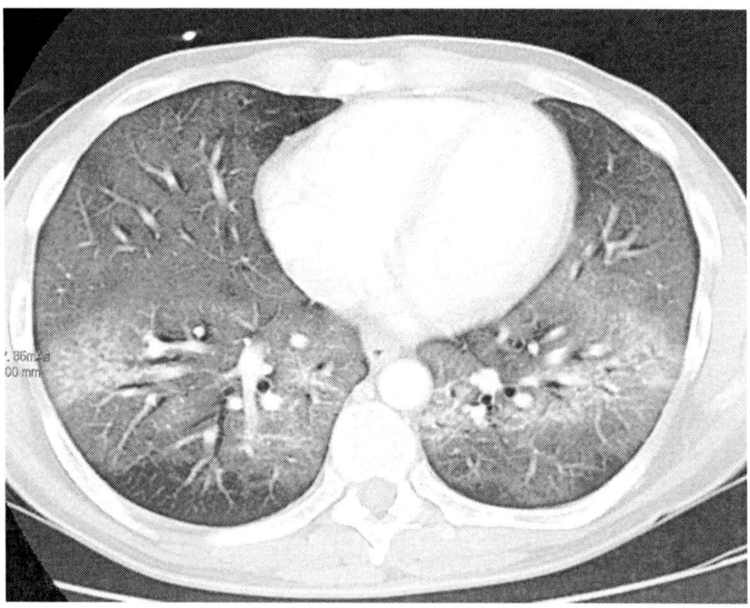

2b

Figure 2. Radiographic findings of Pneumocystis pneumonia. (2a) Chest x-ray of a Pneumocystis pneumonia in a patient with brain neoplasm revealing diffuse infiltrations in both lung fields. (2b) Chest high-resolution CT scan of a patient with renal transplantation showing diffuse ground glass opacities and thickened alveolar septum in both lungs.

Immunorestitution disease (IRD) is defined as an acute symptomatic or paradoxical deterioration of a (most probably) preexisting infection that is temporally related to the recovery of the immune system and it is due to immunopathological damage associated with the reversal of immunosuppressive processes. PcP manifesting as a form of IRD has been described in both HIV and non-HIV immunosuppressed patients [28-30]. Among HIV-infected patients, PcP manifesting acutely during the initiation of HAART is a well-recognized phenomenon [31]. AIDS-related PcP patients seem to be at risk of clinical deterioration due to IRD if antiretroviral therapy is started within one to two weeks after the initiation of treatment for PcP [31,32]. The onset of clinical deterioration is associated with an increase in the CD4 lymphocyte count and a reduction in the HIV viral load [31,32].

In non-HIV immunosuppressed patients, the clinical symptoms of PcP may be unmasked during the reversal of immunosuppression, often at the time when the dose of steroids is tapered or when the endogenous steroid production is reduced [33,34]. Rapid reduction of immunosuppressive therapy has been implicated as a predisposing factor for the development of PcP in non-HIV immunosuppressed patients. In this group of patients, PcP manifesting as IRD often runs an acute and fulminant course, with nonspecific lesions on chest radiographs and high lymphocyte counts. This atypical presentation can delay the diagnosis of PcP if physicians do not have a high index of suspicion [32].

Extrapulmonary manifestations of *P. jirovecii* infection (extrapulmonary pneumocystosis) are distinctly unusual. Extrapulmonary pneumocystosis has been reported primarily among HIV-infected patients, particularly those who receive aerosolized pentamidine for prophylaxis of PcP. Mainly, during the terminal stage of HIV-related disease *Pneumocystis* organisms may disseminate from the lungs to other organs where they induce secondary visceral lesions. However, at times pulmonary infection may not be apparent when extrapulmonary lesions are detected. For HIV-infected patients, extrapulmonary pneumocystosis limited to the choroid layer or ear (external auditory canal or middle ear) has a better prognosis, with good response to specific treatment, than disseminated pneumocystosis in multiple noncontiguous sites. Disseminated pneumocystosis is usually clinically evident, with symptoms related to the affected organs. Lymph nodes, spleen, kidneys, liver, thyroid, and bone marrow are the most commonly infected organs, but microorganisms have also been found in the brain, pancreas, skin, heart, muscle, and other organs [35]. Lesions are frequently nodular and may contain necrotic material or calcification. Extrapulmonary pneumocystosis in solid organs appears on the computed tomography scan as focal, hypodense lesions with well-defined borders and central or peripheral calcification [26]. Non-HIV-associated extrapulmonary pneumocystosis has been rarely reported. In the described cases, disseminated disease often occurred immediately premortem and extrapulmonary pneumocystosis was not clinically evident [35].

In all cases, the clinical diagnosis is complicated because no combination of symptoms, signs, blood chemistries, or radiographic findings is specific of *Pneumocystis* infection. As such, identification of *Pneumocystis* organisms or its DNA in a clinically relevant sample is required to make a diagnosis.

Diagnosis

The single most important diagnostic tool for *Pneumocystis* infection is a high clinical suspicion. In the right clinical setting, an immunosuppressed patient with new onset of dyspnea or new symptoms of pneumonia, with or without radiological findings, should prompt further evaluation, particularly if they are not receiving chemoprophylaxis.

Laboratory Diagnosis of PCP

Microscopic Detection of Pneumocystis

P. jirovecii organisms are usually detected in bronchoalveolar lavage fluids (BALF), induced sputum (IS) samples, or lung biopsy specimens by means of light microscopy (figure 3), immunofluorescence, or molecular methods. No in vitro system for obtaining routinely *Pneumocystis* isolates from patients is available. Using light microscopy, parasites, especially mature cysts, can be detected using phase contrast or Nomarski interference contrast on wet smears. However, microbiologists now detect these parasites on air-dried smears stained by toluidine blue O (TBO), Gomori-Grocott's methenamine silver nitrate (GMS), or methanol-Giemsa methods [36,37].

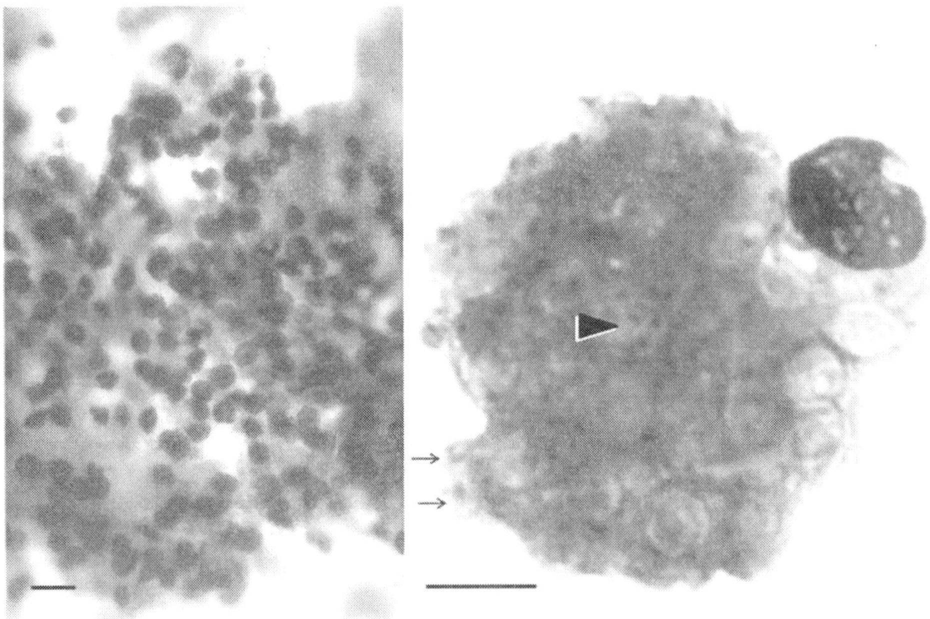

Figure 3. Pneumocystis organisms in cytospin smears of human bronchoalveolar lavage fluid samples. Left: clustered cystic forms stained with Gomori–Grocott's methenamine silver nitrate. Right: Pneumocystis organisms stained with methanol–Giemsa stain: clustered trophic, sporocytic, and cystic forms. A mature cyst containing many spores is quite visible (arrowhead). The cell wall of cystic and sporocytic forms appears as a clear, thin peripheral halo. An alveolar macrophage may also be observed (top right). Bar= 10 µm.

TBO, cresyl violet, and GMS have a good affinity for components of the cyst wall [38]. Thus, TBO stains the cell walls of cystic forms metachromatically in reddish violet and GMS in dark brown. Silver particles deposit on the glucan-rich electron-lucent middle layer of the cyst wall; in contrast, only little silver deposition was recorded in the electron-dense, unique layer of the thin trophic form's cell wall, as shown by ultrastructural studies [39].

TBO or GMS stains facilitate rapid parasite detection, even at low magnification, in all kinds of clinical specimens. However, these dyes also stain the cell wall of yeasts or other fungi. For this reason, a good strategy to identify *Pneumocystis* organisms accurately in clinical specimens is to systematically associate the examination of both TBO- or GMS-stained smears and methanol-Giemsa–stained smears from the same specimen (table 1). Actually, methanol-Giemsa (or other equivalent panoptical Giemsa-like stains) makes it possible, on the one hand, to distinguish *Pneumocystis* organisms from other microorganism and, on the other hand, to identify the different *Pneumocystis* life-cycle stages (figure 3). In fact, Giemsa and other stains with similar cytological affinities, such as Diff Quick or RAL-555, cause the parasite nuclei to stain pinkish purple and the cytoplasm to stain blue [40,41]. They do not stain cystic or sporocytic walls, which appear like a clear peripheral halo around cystic forms. These polychrome stains make it possible accurately to distinguish *Pneumocystis* trophic or cystic forms from other fungi and also from host cells or cell debris. On the whole, the biggest advantage of methanol-Giemsa or Giemsa-like stain methods consists in staining trophic forms and sporocytes (figure 3), which remain unidentified in TBO- or GMS-stained smears [41].

In order to detect *Pneumocystis* organisms in histological sections from lung or other organs, pathologists target usually the cystic forms, since trophic ones are uneasily identifiable in paraffin-embedded tissues. Therefore, they use GMS and, less frequently, TBO staining procedures adapted to tissue sections. Trophic forms can however be identified in epon-embedded semi-thin sections stained with toluidine blue or other stains [41,42]. Furthermore, *Pneumocystis*-specific fluorescein, phosphatase or peroxidase-labeled monoclonal antibodies available from many suppliers may help to identify *Pneumocystis* organisms in BALF, IS or tissue samples (table 1).

Efficiency and cost-effectiveness of the different microscopic stains evoked here vary according to the experience of groups, technical protocols, local incidence of PcP and other factors [43] (table 1). It is generally accepted, however, that association of methods that stain the cystic cell wall (e.g. TBO or GMS) with panoptical techniques (methanol-Giemsa or analogous staining methods) is usually required [44,45]. Moreover, it is usually recognized that specific antibody staining is mainly helpful to detect *Pneumocystis* organisms in non-BALF smears (e.g. IS, expectorated sputum, gastric wash) and to clarify conflicting light microscopic observations [17,46-48]. Finally, it must be remembered that the actual PcP diagnostic currently relies on microscopic detection of *Pneumocystis* cysts and/or trophic forms on stained respiratory samples [17], and that bronchoalveolar lavage is usually regarded as a gold standard procedure, with reported sensitivities ranging from 90% to 98% [49,50].

Table 1. Laboratory diagnostic methods for Pneumocystis pneumonia

Technique	Suitable kind of sample	Needed experience	Sensitivity	Specificity	Advantages	Drawbacks	Recommended combination with:
Microscopy: PC/IC	BALF wet smear	very good	Variable	good	rapidity	needs confirmation by other methods	panoptical stain
GMS/TBO	BALF air-dried cytospin smear or biopsy (histological section)	average	High	average	cost; rapidity	false positive (poor experienced staffs); identifies only the cystic stages	panoptical stain
Panoptical stains*	BALF air-dried cytospin smear	very good	Average	very high	cost; rapidity; identify all Pneumocystis stages	limited sensitivity (poor experienced staffs)	GMS/TBO
FL Mab	BALF, IS or sputum air-dried cytospin smear	good	High	good	good sensitivity/ specificity	cost; time-consuming	-
IP/AP Mab	biopsy (histological section), air-dried cytospin smear	good	Good	good	good specificity	cost; time-consuming	-

PCR	BALF, IS, OW, NPA, biopsy	average	very high	very high	Helpful in HIV-negative patients; rapidity (real-time PCR assays); non-invasive sampling; genotyping	cost; positive in colonized patients	-
BG	serum	average	Good	low	rapidity; post-therapeutic control	positive in other deep fungal infections	other tests
KL-6	serum	average	Good	low	-	positive in other pulmonary infections	
Serum Pneumocystis antibody assay	serum	average	depending on antigen and assay	depending on antigen and assay	helpful in epidemiology studies	positive in people without PcP	other tests

*Giemsa or Giemsa-like stains.

BALF: Bronchoalveolar lavage fluid; BG: serum beta-1,3-glucan; FL Mab: fluorescein-labeled Pneumocystis monoclonal antibody; GMS: Grocott-methenamine silver stain; IP/AP Mab: immuneperoxidase/alkaline-phosphatase labeled monoclonal antibody; IS: induced sputum; PC/IC: phase contrast/interference contrast; TBO; toluidine blue stain. KL-6: Mucin like glycoprotein.

Molecular Detection of Pneumocystis

Many *Pneumocystis* PCR assays were developed in the last two decades. PCR tools were revealed as highly efficacious to amplify *Pneumocystis* DNA from diverse kinds of clinical specimens (BALF, IS, expectorated sputum, oropharyngeal, or nasopharyngeal wash samples, biopsy specimens) (figure 4) [51-56]. In the clinical laboratory, the use of molecular methods is mainly warranted to increase the sensitivity of *P. jirovecii* detection in clinical specimens in order to establish earlier PcP diagnosis, detecting low parasite rates, mainly in non-HIV infected patients with PcP, and detecting *Pneumocystis* DNA in noninvasive samples [54,57] (table 1). Moreover, PCR assays followed by direct sequencing or other strategies were used for typing *Pneumocystis* isolates in order to identify parasite strains and to explore correlation between specific genotypes and virulence, transmissibility or drug susceptibility. PCR, especially nested PCR assays applied to noninvasive samples, have also been used to detect *Pneumocystis* colonization either in susceptible individuals or in apparently healthy people, including healthcare staffs in hospitals [55,58,59].

For PcP diagnosis in humans, conventional or real-time PCR assays based on the amplification of the large subunit of mitochondrial ribosomal DNA (mtLSUrDNA) [51,60] are the most commonly used, but many other sequences have been targeted (Major Surface Glycoprotein, Internal Transcribed Spacers, Thymidylate Synthase, Dihydrofolate Reductase, heat-shock protein 70, etc.) [54,61,62]. Comparative evaluating studies are not easy to perform because of different clinical contexts, sampling methods, laboratory reagents or technical strategies used for DNA extraction, amplification or analysis of results [54].

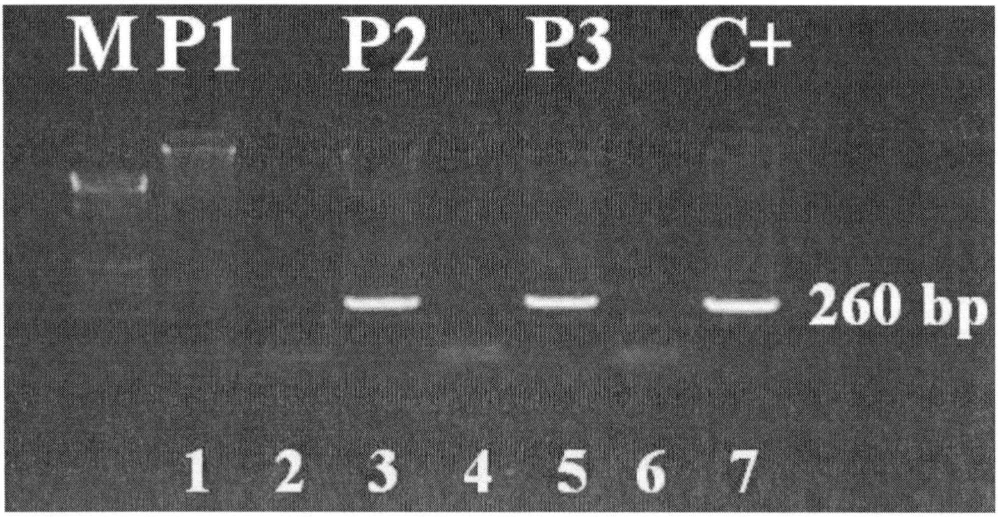

Figure 4. Nested PCR (mtLSU rRNA region) results. M: molecular mass marker. Lane 1 (P1) negative specimen. Lanes 3 and 5 (P2, P3) positive specimens of oral wash in cystic fibrosis patients. Lane 7 (C+) positive control. Lanes 2, 4 and 6 negative controls (water).

In general, conventional, or real-time *Pneumocystis* PCR assays, have represented a significant advance in PcP laboratory diagnosis. Actually, highly sensitive and specific PCR tools, especially real-time PCR assays, improved the clinical diagnosis of PcP allowing an accurate, early diagnosis of *Pneumocystis* infection [54], which should lead to a decreased duration from onset of symptoms to treatment. This period has a recognized impact on prognosis since PcP-associated respiratory failure requiring mechanic ventilation entails significant mortality [63]. In addition, PCR assay may reveal PcP in patients with negative microscopic test. For instance, among 62 HIV-negative patients with clinical PcP diagnosed in the Lille University Hospital between 1998 and 2001, 30 patients (48%) had positive PCR results with negative microscopic tests [64].

Notably, molecular techniques play a significant role when they are applied to noninvasive specimens as IS, oropharyngeal wash (OW, obtained by gargling 10 ml of 0.9% NaCl for >60 seconds) [57,65-67] or nasopharyngeal aspirates (NPA) [68]. When DNA sequences used as primers or probes have been adequately defined, the analytical specificity of *Pneumocystis*-PCR assays applied to noninvasive or to BALF samples should usually be 100% [54,61,66]. With regard to sensitivity, *Pneumocystis*-mtLSUrDNA PCR showed high analytical sensitivity for the detection of *Pneumocystis* organisms on BALF samples from AIDS patients, with a detection threshold of 0.5–1 organism/μl^{-1} [61]. The sensitivity of PCR assays applied to OW (or other noninvasive samples) is certainly lower (<80%) [60,65,69] than that of PCR on BALF samples (>95%) [68]. However, OW can be easily repeated in order to monitor the evolution of infection and, potentially, the therapeutic response [60].

A significant problem of *Pneumocystis* PCR assays is raised by *Pneumocystis* colonization [70]. Actually, a positive PCR result associated with a negative microscopic test may result from either *Pneumocystis* colonization or PcP. In common practice, this difficulty is often solved with careful clinical, radiological and laboratory assessment of the patient's pathological condition, as is usually done with other infectious diseases, especially when their agents are opportunistic pathogens. However, the alternative of quantifying parasite rates was also explored [71]. Thus, a quantitative real-time PCR assay that targeted the *Pneumocystis* Major Surface Glycoprotein (MSG) multigene family was applied to OW samples, and revealed significant differences between PcP patients and *Pneumocystis* colonized subjects in the number of MSG copies. The authors suggested a cutoff value of 50 MSG gene fragment copies/tube for distinguishing between the two conditions [71]. However, quantitative PCR results seemed difficult to use in the field. The main problem was the inability to control the volume of the sample. Another difficulty relates to the kind of patients. Actually, it seems difficult to apply the same cutoff to AIDS patients, patients with other underlying diseases, or individuals receiving chemoprophylaxis against *Pneumocystis*.

There is no formal agreement about an unequivocal definition of *Pneumocystis* colonization. The notion may however be characterized by clinical and experimental observations. In clinical practice, the diagnosis of *Pneumocystis* colonization or subclinical carriage is usually retained when *Pneumocystis* DNA is detected by PCR methods in respiratory samples from immunodepressed or immunocompetent subjects without symptoms or signs of *Pneumocystis* infection, and who do not progress to PcP [72]. In these subjects, *Pneumocystis* organisms are only exceptionally detected by microscopy [73]. Interestingly, recent experimental data strengthened the biological significance of *Pneumocystis* colonization [74]. They demonstrated that *Pneumocystis* organisms can replicate in the lungs of immunocompetent carriers, stimulate an antibody response and be efficiently transmitted by airborne route to either naive immunocompetent hosts, who will develop a primary infection, or to immunosuppressed hosts, who may then develop PcP [74]. In addition, there is evidence to suggest that beyond PcP, *Pneumocystis* colonization may induce local or systemic inflammation, a condition that could aggravate chronic pulmonary diseases. For instance, *P. jirovecii* pulmonary carriage in patients with chronic obstructive pulmonary disease (COPD) could favor the progression of this disease [72,75], which is a major cause of death worldwide [76].

Efforts have been made to associate specific *P. jirovecii* genotypes with virulence, drug susceptibility or other medically important biological properties of parasite strains. Some studies reported some correlation between polymorphism and clinical features [65,77,78]. Polymorphism of internal transcribed spacer (ITS1/ITS2) sequences was quite frequently used and more than 30 ITS1 genotypes and 40 ITS2 genotypes with more than 90 haplotypes (combinations of ITS1 and ITS2 types) have been reported [79]. It was shown that a high proportion of ITS recombinants, detected under standard conditions, would be chimeras generated during the genotyping process mainly during elongation [80]. However, this difficulty could be overcome by combining several measures (adding a proofreading polymerase, extending the elongation time, increasing melting temperature, decreasing the number of cycles) [80].

Most polymorphism studies targeted mutations of the *P. jirovecii* dihydropteroate synthase (DHPS) gene, which could potentially be linked with sulfa resistance. Regarding this issue, and since effective *P. jirovecii* culture systems are unavailable, several groups have assessed putative trimethoprim-sulfamethoxazole drug resistance by detecting *Pneumocystis* DHPS mutations. Indeed nonsynonymous DHPS point mutations at nucleotide positions 165 and 171 entail an amino acid change at positions 55 (Thr to Ala) and/or 57 (Pro to Ser) [81]. Such mutations confer resistance to sulfa drugs in other organisms, including *Escherichia coli*, *Streptococcus pneumoniae* and *Plasmodium falciparum*. The *P. jirovecii* DHPS mutant form has also been shown to be more resistant to sulfamethoxazole in a *Saccharomyces cerevisiae* model [82], but it is still uncertain if *Pneumocystis* DHPS mutations lead to drug resistance in patients [83,84]. Such mutations were shown to be associated with the use of trimethoprim-sulfamethoxazole or dapsone (two DHPS inhibitors), the duration of sulfa or dapsone prophylaxis and with geographic areas in which sulfamethoxazole or dapsone were commonly used for PcP prophylaxis [84-86]. However, results of studies searching specifically to establish an association between the presence of *P. jirovecii* DHPS mutations and clinical outcomes, such as treatment failure or death, are contradictory [84,87-91]. Outstandingly, most PcP patients carrying *P. jirovecii* isolates with DHPS mutations responded well to trimethoprim-sulfamethoxazole (TMP-SMX)treatment and survived probably because these mutations may confer a low-level of resistance to sulfa-drugs that is overcome by high drug concentration achieved in lung tissues by sulfamethoxazole [84,92,93].

Other Laboratory Diagnostic Methods

a) Beta-D-glucan assay

β-1,3-glucan (BG) is the main structural component of the cell wall of all fungi, including *Pneumocystis* cysts [94]. Interestingly, high serum BG levels have been reported in patients with PcP [95-97]. Consistently, such levels decreased with effective anti-*Pneumocystis* treatment [96]. Serum BG appeared therefore as a good marker of *Pneumocystis* infection.

The potential utility of this assay was illustrated in a retrospective case-control study of 295 patients with suspected PcP comparing BG with microscopic examination of BAL. The BG assay had a sensitivity of 92% and a specificity of 86% for detecting PcP for a cut-off level of 31.1 pg/ml [98].

In a recent study, it has been observed that BG levels in non-HIV patients with PcP are lower than in HIV patients. This could be attributed to the fact that HIV patients have greater numbers of microorganisms than non-HIV patients [97].

However, BG levels could not be correlated with PcP prognosis, and false positive results could exceed more than 30% [97]. False positive results were reported in patients undergoing bacterial septicemia, hemodialysis with cellulose dialysis membranes, treatment with immunoglobulin, glucan-containing antitumor drugs, amoxicillin-clavulanate, piperacillin-tazobactam or contact with gauze or surgical sponges containing BG [99]. Furthermore, since invasive fungal infections also induce an increase of serum BG, the test should often be associated with laboratory assays aiming at detecting such infections [95]. At least four BG assays allowing assessing serum BG levels in clinical laboratories are available: Fungitec G, Wako and B-G Star, which are used in Japan; Fungitell, which is used in Europe and USA [99].

These preliminary studies suggest that in the right clinical setting serum BG may provide a useful noninvasive diagnostic adjunct for patients with *Pneumocystis* infection. However, additional information is necessary to address the general specificity of BG in diagnosing PcP versus other fungal infections in diverse immune-suppressed patient populations and to differentiate among patients with PcP and patients with *Pneumocystis* colonization.

b) *S*-adenosylmethionine (SAM)

Some observations suggested that S-adenosylmethionine (SAM), which is a universal methyl donor synthesized from methionine and ATP by SAM synthetase, could stimulate *Pneumocystis* in vitro growth [100]. Since SAM was depleted from both the culture medium and the plasma of rats with PcP, it was hypothesized that *Pneumocystis* cells could scavenge SAM from host fluids due to the lack of SAM synthetase [100]. Consistently, plasma SAM levels were found to be low in patients with PcP and to increase gradually with treatment [101,102]. These findings strengthened the idea of using plasma SAM levels as a non-invasive PcP diagnostic method. However, recent data showed that SAM-related issues could be more complex than previously thought. Firstly, differences in SAM levels between laboratories could be influenced by the method of measurement. Thus, Wang and colleagues using Chromatography Tandem Mass Spectrometry found generally higher plasma SAM levels than those reported before [103]. The same group was unable to distinguish patients with acute PcP from the ones without PcP based on plasma SAM levels, though these levels increased significantly with effective anti-*Pneumocystis* treatment. Indeed, the concern needs to be further explored because fasting status, dietary intake of methionine, and other medications can affect plasma SAM concentration [103]. Secondly, and contrary to the results of previous works [100], *P. carinii*, *P. murina* and *P. jirovecii* have genes that encoded SAM synthetase (Sam1) [104]. Moreover, the corresponding *Sam1* mRNA is transcribed, and the protein, which is enzymatically active, was immuno-localized in *P. murina* cells. Such data suggest strongly that the *Pneumocystis* species do not depend on an exogenous source of SAM to survive [104].

c) KL-6

KL-6 is a mucin-like glycoprotein expressed on type II pneumocytes and bronchiolar epithelial cells. This serological marker has been found in elevated levels in several studies in patients with PcP. However, the reported false-positive rate and level of detection were not as good as for the BG assay [97,98]. Recent investigations indicant that JKL-6 is more a generalized marker for alveolar epithelial injury [105] and can also be detected in non-fungal infections such as *Legionella*, severe tuberculosis and respiratory syncythial virus bronchiolitis, and even in noninfectious interstitial lung disease [106-108]. Therefore, the KL-6 elevation in PcP is thought to be related to lung damage and regeneration of epithelium lining and cannot be used as a specified marker of *Pneumocystis* infection.

d) Serological tests

Serum antibody detection constitutes an adjunctive strategy currently used to diagnose systemic fungal infections, even in immunodepressed patients. However, this strategy was rarely used for PcP diagnosis because healthy subjects frequently have significant levels of the serum *Pneumocystis* antibody. Moreover, the antibody response against *Pneumocystis* infection is currently highly variable and the results reported by diverse groups are contradictory [109]. In contrast, *Pneumocystis* antibody assays, especially those using recombinant *Pneumocystis* antigens, constitute an interesting tool in epidemiology [110].

Management Strategies for PCP

There is no universally agreed approach on the initial management of patients with suspected PcP. Many institutions treat patients with suspected PcP empirically, while others pursue a definitive microbiological diagnosis [63]. In the absence of prospective studies comparing various management and diagnostic strategies, the specific approach to a patient with suspected PcP is often based on the incidence of PcP and clinician and institutional preferences and experiences [17,63]. Since PcP can be rapidly progressive and the mortality rate remains high, particularly among non-HIV immunosuppressed patients, early therapy is essential [8-10].

Identification of patients having mild, moderate or severe PcP disease guides the choice of drug for the treatment, as well as to decide if adjuvant corticosteroids are indicated (table 2) [111]. In AIDS-related PcP, the typical duration of therapy is at least 21 days because of the risk for relapse with shorter treatment duration. However, in patients with PcP without HIV-infection two weeks of treatment is usually adequate, even though treatment should be individualized and extended if recovery is prolonged [10,23,112,113]. There are no randomized trial data indicating when specific anti-*Pneumocystis* therapy should be modified because of inadequate response [114,115]. In the absence of corticosteroid therapy, early and reversible deterioration within the first 3–5 days of therapy is typical. Patients generally improved after 4 to 8 days of therapy. Therefore, changes in treatment due to lack of efficacy should rarely be made prior to 4 to 8 days and noninfectious processes, as congestive heart failure or pulmonary emboli, or concurrent infections should be ruled out previously [112,113].

Table 2. Grading of severity of Pneumocystis pneumonia

	Mild	Moderate	Severe
Symptoms and signs	Dyspnoea on exertion, with or without cough and sweats	Dyspnoea on minimal exertion and occasionally at rest. Cough and fever	Dyspnoea and tachypnoea at rest. Persistent fever and cough
Arterial oxygen tension (PaO2) at rest	> 11.0 kPa (82.7 mmHg)	8.0 to 11.0 kPa (60-82.7 mmHg)	< 8.0 kPa (60 mmHg)
Arterial oxygen saturation (SaO2) at rest	> 96%	91 to 96%	< 91%
Chest radiograph	Normal, or minor perihiliar shadowing	Diffuse interstitial shadowing	Extension interstitial shadowing with or without diffuse alveolar shadowing

Modified of Miller RF, et al. J. Antimicrob. Chemother. 1996; 37 (Suppl B): 33-53 [135

Although the overall prognosis of patients whose degree of hypoxemia requires intensive care unit (ICU) admission or mechanical ventilation remains poor, survival in up to 50% of patients requiring ventilatory support has been reported. Patients with reasonable functional status and severe PcP should be offered ICU admission or mechanical ventilation [112].

Treatment

The recommended treatment of PcP has remained unchanged for many years, being Co-trimoxazole, an association of trimethoprim and sulfamethoxazole, the drug of choice as first line of treatment. Regarding which agent is preferred for the second line of choice, data are limited (table 3).

Drug related toxicities are increasing in HIV-infected patients and organ transplant recipients. Because of the potential for additive or synergistic toxicities associated with anti-*Pneumocystis* and antiretroviral therapies, certain health-care providers delay initiation of HAART until after the completion of anti-*Pneumocystis* therapy, or until at least 2 weeks after initiating anti-*Pneumocystis* therapy, despite some suggestion of potential benefit of early HAART in the treatment of patients with AIDS-related opportunistic infections [112,116]. In order to correctly manage PcP, it is important to distinguish between progressive PcP, drug toxicity, and concomitant infection if clinical deterioration is detected.

Table 3. Drug therapy for treatment of Pneumocystis pneumonia in adults according to severity

	Moderate to severe Pneumocystis pneumonia		
Therapeutic use	Drug	Dose	Route
First line	Trimethoprim-Sulfamethoxazole	15-20 mg/Kg daily divided into 3 or 4 doses 75-100 mg/Kg daily divided into 3 or 4 doses	Intravenous
Second line	Primaquine plus Clindamycin	30 mg daily 600-900 mg three times daily	Oral Intravenous
Second line	Pentamidine	4 mg/Kg daily (3 mg/Kg if toxicities)	Intravenous
Salvage therapy	Trimetrexate plus Leucovorin	45 mg/m^2 daily 20 mg/m^2 four times daily	Intravenous Intravenous or oral
Adjunctive therapy	Prednisone Methylprednisolone	Days 1–5: 80 mg daily divided into 2 doses Days 6–10: 40 mg daily Days 11–21: 20 mg daily 75% of prednisone dose	Oral Intravenous
	Mild to moderate Pneumocystis pneumonia		
First line	Trimethoprim-Sulfamethoxazole	15-20 mg/Kg daily divided into 3 doses 75-100 mg/Kg daily divided into 3 doses	Oral
Second line	Dapsone plus Trimethoprim	100 mg daily 15-20 mg/Kg daily divided into 3 doses	Oral Oral or intravenous
Second line	Primaquine plus Clindamycin	15-30 mg daily 300-450 mg 3 or 4 times daily	Oral Oral
Second line	Atovaquone	750 mg two times daily	Oral with food

Trimethoprim-Sulfamethoxazole (TMP-SMX)

TMP and SMX target sequential steps in the folate synthesis pathway. TMP inhibits dihydrofolate reductase and SMX inhibits dihydrotperoate synthetase. TMP-SMX is the treatment of choice for PcP in all patients who tolerate this drug, and it achieves the most rapid clinical response of the anti-*Pneumocystis* agents [112,117]. The recommended dose of TMP-SMX for adults (or children aged > 2 months) is 15 to 20 mg/kg/day of TMP and 75 to 100 mg/kg/day of SMX intravenously every 6 or 8 hours. With renal dysfunction, dosing must be reduced. The bioavailability of TMP-SMX from oral therapy is comparable to parenteral administration [112,118].

Patients, who have PcP despite the use of TMP-SMX prophylaxis, are usually successfully treated with TMP-SMX. In this way, the presence of mutations in the DHPS gene of *P. jirovecii* has been associated with resistance to sulfa drugs, although the clinical outcome is uncertain [84,91,119]. Drug related toxicities from TMP-SMX are greater than that from therapy with other anti-*Pneumocystis* agents. The side effects of TMP-SMX are: rash (30-55%), (including Stevens-Johnson syndrome), fever (30-40%), leukopenia (30-40%), hepatitis (20%), thrombocytopenia (15%), azotemia (1-5%), and hyperkaliemia [120-122]. Nephrotoxicity occurs frequently in the renal transplantation recipient receiving full-dose of TMP-SMX. Liver transplant recipients are particularly susceptible to TMP-SMX toxicity. Leucovorin to prevent myelosuppression is not recommended because of its uncertain efficacy and higher rate of failure [112].

Pentamidine

Pentamidine is an aromatic diamidine that has broad-spectrum anti-protozoal activity. This drug inhibits metabolism of *P* amino benzoic acid, interferes with anaerobic glycolysis, inhibits oxidative phosphorylation, and impairs nucleic acid and protein synthesis. It was the first drug reported to treat PcP successfully and subsequent reports have confirmed the efficacy of intravenous pentamidine. Although intravenous pentamidine has been recommended as the main alternative to TMP-SMX for moderate to severe PcP [121], a recent study has found a greater risk of death when pentamidine was used as first and second-line therapy for HIV-associated PcP as compared with TMP-SMX and clindamycin-primaquine [117]. These findings could be due to toxicities related to pentamidine and the absence of an antibacterial effect, in contrast to TMP-SMX or clindamycin-primaquine, which might act against concomitant bacterial co-infection [117].

Pentamidine for children and adults is administered once a day at 4 mg/kg (maximum 300 mg daily) intravenously, infused slowly 1 to 2 hr in 5% glucose; due to its toxicity, the dose can be reduced to 3 mg/kg. Aerosolized pentamidine should not be used because of limited efficacy and more frequent relapse, and intramuscular administration is not used due to the related complications [123]. Side effects of pentamidine include azotemia, pancreatitis, hypo- or hyperglycemia, pancytopenia, electrolyte abnormalities, cardiac dysrhythmia and renal dysfunction [123,124]. Pentamidine should be avoided in pancreas transplant recipients due to the potential for islet cell necrosis.

Clindamycin-Primaquine

Clindamycin is a lincosamide antibiotic used to treat infections with anaerobic bacteria but can also be used to treat some protozoan diseases. Primaquine is an 8-aminoquinoline anti-protozoan agent. This combination is effective in adult patients with mild to moderate PcP, but data for children are not available [125,126]. Clindamycin is given at 600 to 900 mg intravenously or 300-450 mg orally every 6 to 8 hours and primaquine is given at 15 to 30 mg/day given orally. Clindamycin component can be administered intravenously in severe cases; primaquine is only available orally. Recently, clindamycin-primaquine appeared superior to pentamidine as second-line therapy for PcP in patients failing or developing toxicity with TMP-SMX [117]. Side effects of clindamycin include rash, anemia, neutropenia and the development of *Clostridium difficile* colitis. The main toxicity of primaquine is methemoglobinemia, thus, patients should be tested for glucose-6-phosphate dehydrogenase deficiency before administration of primaquine [113].

Dapsone

Dapsone is a sulfone drug that inhibits DHPS and it is used as an alternative therapeutic regimen for mild-to-moderate PcP. Dapsone must be taken with TMP [127]. Although this association might have similar efficacy and fewer side effects than TMP-SMX, it is less recommended due to the number of pills. The dosage of dapsone for adolescents and adults is 100 mg orally once daily (among children aged < 13 years, 2 mg/kg/day). The dosage of TMP for children and adults taken orally is 15 mg/kg/day divided into three doses [112,118]. The most common adverse effects associated to dapsone are methemoglobinemia and hemolysis, especially in those with glucose-6-phosphate dehydrogenase deficiency. Thus, patients should be tested for glucose-6-phosphate dehydrogenase deficiency [113].

Atovaquone

Atovaquone is a unique naphthoquinone that targets the cytochome B complex and, thus, inhibits mitochondrial electron transport. This drug was developed clinically in the 1990s and it is available only as oral agent. It is used as a second-line agent for treatment of mild to moderate PcP if TMP-SMX cannot be used. The standard dosing regimen for adults is atovaquone 750 mg orally twice a day with food for increasing gastrointestinal absorption (30-40 mg/kg/day for children < 3 months and > 24 months of age; between 3-24 months of age, 45 mg/kg/day are required) [118,127]. Mutations of the cytochrome *b* gene have occurred in atovaquone-resistant isolates of *Pneumocystis*, but the clinical significance of gene mutations has not been determined [129]. The advantages of atovaquone include oral administration and fewer side effects. Disadvantages are its high cost and its bioavailability, although it has been improved with the micronized suspension formulation [128]. The most frequently reported adverse effects are rash, nausea, diarrhea, elevation of liver enzyme levels and headache. Atovaquone does not cause bone marrow suppression [113].

Trimetrexate

Trimetrexate is an analogue of methotrexate that is an inhibitor of dihydrofolate reductase, and *in vitro* it is 1500 times more potent than trimethoprim [130,131]. This drug is effective for treating PcP but is available only in an intravenous formulation. Because this drug also inhibits human folate metabolism, leucovorin must be administered concomitantly to prevent cytopenias [113]. A clinical trial showed that trimetrexate is less effective but better tolerated than TMP-SMX against AIDS-related PcP [132]. Trimetrexate with folinic acid have been approved for use in patients with moderately severe PcP, however, it is no longer available commercially. The dosage recommended for treatment of PcP is trimetrexate, 45 mg/m^2 intravenously once daily, plus leucovorin 20 mg/m^2 orally or intravenously four times daily [132]. Leucovorin therapy must extend for 72 hours past the last dose of trimetrexate. For adults, trimetrexate may alternatively be dosed on a mg/kg basis, depending on the patient's body weight: <50 kg, 1.5 mg/kg; 50-80 kg, 1.2 mg/kg, and >80 kg, 1.0 mg/kg. Also, leucovorin may be dosed on a mg/kg basis (<50 kg, 0.6 mg/kg, and >50 kg 0.5 mg/kg) administered every 6 hours. Despite the suggestion that leucovorin impairs the efficacy of TMP-SMX, there is no indication that the coadministration of leucovorin impairs the efficacy of trimetrexate for PcP [113]. In some cases, trimetrexate plus leucovorin could be used as salvage treatment for PcP [133].

Adjunctive Therapies

The use of corticosteroids may reduce pulmonary inflammation response caused by the lysis of *Pneumocystis* in the lung after initiating treatment of PcP. Corticosteroids have been related with a significant benefit in terms of preventing deterioration in oxygenation in the first seven days of therapy, mortality, and reduction of intubations in AIDS patients [134]. Corticosteroids are indicated in HIV-infected patients with a moderate-to-severe PcP, who have hypoxemia (the partial pressure of arterial oxygen less than 70 mm Hg with the patient breathing room air or an alveolar-arteriolar gradient greater than 35). In these cases, corticosteroids should be administered as early as possible within 72 hours after starting anti-*Pneumocystis* therapy [18,112]. Recommended doses are shown in table 3.

In non-HIV infected patients with PcP there are no randomized clinical trials about the use of adjunctive corticosteroids and data are far less clear. Moreover, non-HIV immunocompromised patients constitute a heterogeneous group of patients and most of them have been on corticosteroid at the time they developed PcP. Therefore, the recommendations of adjunctive corticosteroids therapy in non-HIV patient must be individualized. In patients with severe PcP a dose of 60 mg or more of prednisone daily resulted in a better outcome than lower doses of prednisone [135].

Novel Agents

Novel agents undergoing clinical investigation include echinocandins and pneumocandins, which target synthesis of beta 1,3 glucan, a cell wall compound of Pneumocystis and other fungi.

The sordarin family, probably the most active anti-*Pneumocystis* molecules, inhibits protein synthesis in fungi by stabilizing the ribosome/EF2 complex. This mode of action contrasts with a typical antifungal, which targets the cell membrane. Some sordarin derivatives have shown excellent in-vitro and in-animal model activities against a wide range of pathogenic fungi which include *Pneumocystis,* but until now, no clinical trials have been started [136,137].

Caspofungin is an echinochandin that acts on the cell wall by inhibiting β-1,3-glucan synthesis and it has been approved for several fungal infections such as the *Candida* and *Aspergillus* species. Caspofungin has shown activity against *Pneumocystis* in experimental animal models and it has strong activity on cyst forms and weak activity on trophic forms [138]. Because TMP-SMX affects only the trophic forms, it has been suggested that the association of TMP-SMX and caspofungin, by fully inhibiting the organism life cycle, may provide a synergistic activity against *Pneumocystis*. Cases of PcP have been reported where the association of caspofungin and TMP-SMX achieved a complete cure of PcP [139,140]. However, this promising therapeutic approach needs to be assessed by controlled clinical trials.

Prognosis

Despite treatment, mortality from PcP still remains high. Several studies highlight that mortality rates are declining in patients with PcP. However, in other studies, PcP has remained the leading cause of death among those not receiving or failing to comply with HAART or PcP prophylaxis. Predictors of mortality include older age, recent injection drug use, increased total bilirrubin, low serum albumin, and alveolar-arterial oxygen gradient >50 mm Hg [141.

Non-HIV patients present more acutely with fulminate respiratory failure associated with fever and dry cough and frequently require mechanical ventilation. Most studies demonstrate a worse survival (51-80%) in non-HIV patients compared with AIDS patients (86-92%) [142]. As PcP is a severe infection with a high mortality rate, prevention is essential in the groups at risk.

Prophylaxis Regimens for PCP

Many studies have demonstrated that PcP can largely be prevented by administration of chemoprophylaxis to susceptible individuals [11,143-146]. According with the American Thoracic Society recommendations both patients infected with HIV and non-HIV immunosuppressed patients need to receive prophylaxis to prevent disease depending on specific risks to the patient's immune system [147]. Recommendations for chemoprophylaxis should be based on weighing the efficacy against the risk of adverse events, the risk of developments of antimicrobial resistance, and the cost of the intervention [10]. Medications recommended for chemoprophylaxis against PcP are listed in table 4.

Primary Prophylaxis

The majority of recommendations are based on studies performed in HIV-infected patients. Guidelines recommend starting primary prophylaxis against PcP in HIV-infected adolescents and adults, including pregnant patients, and patients under HAART, when the CD4 cell count is less than 200 cells/mm^3 or the patient has a history of oropharyngeal candidiasis. Patients with a CD4 cell percentage of <14% or a history of an AIDS-defining illness should be considered for chemoprophylaxis [112]. Prophylaxis recommendations for HIV-infected children are age-based. Chemoprophylaxis should be provided for children 6 years or older based on adults guidelines, for children aged 1 to 5 years if CD4 counts are less than 500 cells/mm^3 or CD4 percentage is less than 15%, and for all HIV-infected infants younger than 12 months [116].

Table 4. Prophylaxis regimens for Pneumocystis pneumonia

Drug	Dose for adults	Dose for children	Route	Comments
Trimethoprim-Sulfamethoxazole	160/800 mg (DS tablet) per day or 3 times per week 80/400 mg (SS tablet) per day	150/750 mg/m^2 body surface area (max: 320/1600 mg) as single or 2 divided doses 3 times per week	Oral	First choice Weekly regimen is recommended if daily therapy in not tolerated
Dapsone	100 mg per day	2 mg/Kg body weight (max: 100 g) per day 4 mg/Kg body weight (max: 200 g) per week	Oral	Alternative choice Ensure patient does not have Glucose-6 phosphate dehydrogenase deficiency
Pentamidine	300 mg per month	300 mg per month (aged ≥ 5 years)	Aerosol	Alternative choice
Atovaquone	1500 mg per day	30-45 mg/Kg body weight according to age per day	Oral	Alternative choice Take with high-fat meals for maximal absorption
Dapsona + Pyrimethamine + Leucovorin	50 mg per day 50 mg per week 25 mg per week		Oral Oral Oral	Alternative choice Ensure patient does not have Glucose-6 phosphate dehydrogenase deficiency Effective in preventing toxoplasmosis
Dapsona + Pyrimethamine + Leucovorin	200 mg per week 75 mg per week 25 mg per week		Oral Oral Oral	Alternative choice Ensure patient does not have Glucose-6 phosphate dehydrogenase deficiency Effective in preventing toxoplasmosis

Although immunosuppressed HIV-negative patient studies about PcP prophylaxis are limited, a meta-analysis has recently confirmed that prophylaxis with TMP-SMX significantly reduced PcP infections and PcP-related mortality in these patients [143]. Daily systemic administration of corticosteroid is the second most common reason for developing PcP after HIV infection [148-150]. For this reason, administration of chemoprophylaxis to patients who are receiving at least 20 mg of prednisone per day for at least one month has been suggested [10,24]. However, this approach would unnecessarily expose patients to drug side-effects and could potentially encourage drug resistance. As an alternative, it has been suggested that a CD4 cell count of less than 200 cells/mm^3 might indicate the use of PcP prophylaxis in patients who are receiving long-term corticosteroid treatment, although this test is not nearly as sensitive or specific as it is in HIV-infected individuals [149]. In this sense, CD4 cell count could be monitored to determine when to introduce a primary chemoprophylaxis:

- after one month of immunosuppression in patients who are in treatment with steroid dosage greater than 15 mg prednisolone or equivalent per day,
- corticosteroid treatment proposed for more than 3 months or
- total lymphocyte count less than 600 cells/mm^3

However, prospective investigation is required to validate this preventive strategy [10,149].

For non-HIV immunosuppressed patients, there is no reliable laboratory marker for susceptibility. In fact, the benefit of chemoprophylaxis should be balanced with the risk of severe adverse events, and depends on the attack rate of PcP [10,150]. In this sense, it becomes clear that chemoprophylaxis for PcP should be considered when the risk for PcP in adults is higher than 3.5% (among children a much lower risk would probably warrant prophylaxis because adverse events are infrequent) and continued as long as the immunosuppressive condition remains active [143]. Such rates of risk are seen in recipients of solid organ or allogeneic bone marrow during the first 6 months after transplant or after treatment of rejection episodes and, for the latter, throughout the period of immune-suppression, as well as in patients with acute lymphoblastic leukemia and Wegener granulomatosis [143,144]. Available data have led experts to recommend prophylaxis in patients with connective tissue diseases who receive chronic corticosteroid therapy combined with another immunosuppressive drug as well as in patients with systemic lupus erythematosus or Wegener granulomatosis during the first year of treatment, particularly when they have lymphopenia or renal failure [10].

TMP-SMX is the recommended prophylactic agent in both HIV-infected and uninfected immunosuppressed patients, because of its high efficacy, relative safety, low cost, and broad antimicrobial spectrum [10,11,112,144]. TMP–SMX is also effective in preventing *Toxoplasma gondi, Isospora belli, Cyclospora cayetanensis* and some bacterial infections such as, *Streptococcus pneumoniae*, *Salmonella*, *Haemophilus*, *Staphylococcus,* and common gram-negative gastrointestinal and urinary pathogens [11]. Either one single-strength tablet daily or one double-strength tablet daily are the preferred regimens, but the first regimen might be better tolerated than the second [112]. An alternative can be one double-strength tablet three times per week [10,112]. TMP-SMX at a dose of one double-strength tablet daily confers cross-protection against toxoplasmosis and selected common respiratory bacterial infections. Lower doses of TMP-SMX also likely confer such protection [112,144].

For patients who have an adverse reaction that is not life threatening, prophylaxis with TMP-SMX should be reinstituted. These patients might better tolerate reintroduction of the drug with a gradual increase in dose or reintroduction of TMP-SMX at a reduced dose or frequency [112]. If TMP-SMX is not tolerated, a second choice would be dapsone given 100 mg daily, dapsone 50 mg daily plus pyrimethamine 50 mg weekly plus leucovorin 25 mg weekly or dapsone 200 plus pyrimethamine 75 mg plus leucovorin 25 mg weekly, aerosolized pentamidine 300 mg monthly administered by an ultrasonic or jet-nebulizer, and atovaquone

1500 mg daily [11,112]. Dapsone is effective and inexpensive but associated with more serious adverse effects than atovaquone [146]. Atovaquone is effective, safe and it is effective against *Toxoplasma gondii* but it is more expensive [11]. The widespread concept that TMP-SMX is contraindicated for prophylaxis in patients treated with methotrexate might be obsolete because the safety of one single-strength tablet daily or one double-strength tablet thrice weekly has been proved in clinical studies [151,152]. However, these patients need to receive folate supplementation, and blood counts and liver-function tests should be closely monitored [10].

Primary prophylaxis should be discontinued for HIV-infected adult and adolescent patients who have responded to HAART with an increase in CD4 counts higher than 200 cells/mm^3 during more than 3 months [153]. Prophylaxis should be reintroduced if the CD4 cell count decreases to less than 200 cells/mm^3. Concerning immunosuppressed non-HIV-infected patients, data are limited and the optimal duration of chemoprophylaxis is still undecided, although probably the length of prophylaxis should continue as long as the immunosuppressive conditions remains active [10,12,150].

Secondary Prophylaxis

HIV-infected adult and adolescent patients who have developed previous episodes of PcP should receive secondary prophylaxis [18]. Chemoprophylaxis should be discontinued for adult and adolescent patients when the CD4 cell count increases to more than 200 cells/mm^3 for a period of 3 months because of HAART [153]. Prophylaxis should be reintroduced if the CD4 count decreases again to less than 200 cells/mm^3. If PcP recurs at a CD4 count higher than 200 cells/mm^3, continuing PcP prophylaxis for life would be prudent [112].

The risk for recurrence of PcP is undefined in non-HIV immunosuppressed patients and recommendations of secondary prophylaxis have not been established. Alternatives would be to monitor patients closely in order to detect any recurrence or to place patients on secondary chemoprophylaxis throughout the period of susceptibility as long as the immunosuppressive condition persists [10].

Conclusion

Pneumocystis jirovecii is an atypical fungus that causes PcP in HIV-infected individuals and immunosuppressed patients. PcP is today still a major cause of morbidity and mortality among immunocompromised persons, especially those with AIDS, and constitutes a worldwide problem to public health. While the incidence of PcP among HIV infected individuals has decreased in developed countries, the prevalence of AIDS-related PcP in developing countries remains high and poorly controlled. Currently, with the rising number of patients receiving immunosuppressive therapies for malignancies, allogeneic organ transplantations and autoimmune diseases, PcP is being recognized more and more in non-HIV-immunosuppressed individuals in developed countries. The epidemiology of this infection is only beginning to be understood. The accumulating evidence suggests that *P. jirovecii* is a highly infectious organism with low virulence that takes advantage of hosts as temporary reservoirs of infection. In this sense, colonization with *P. jirovecii* (that is infection without disease) has recently gained attention as an important issue for understanding the complete cycle of human *Pneumocystis* infection. The clinical presentation in HIV-infected patients may differ from that in other immunosuppressed patients and its diagnosis continues to be challenging. Clinicians must be familiar with its presentation and management because mild cases are sometimes difficult to diagnose. Co-trimoxazole is the most effective medication for its prevention and treatment but other alternative medications are also available. Future clinical research should also include studying the transmission and epidemiology of PcP in populations worldwide, improving the diagnosis of PcP, improving regimens for prophylaxis and treatment in various patient populations, and determining the significance of the DHPS mutations in various populations and in different geographic locations. Furthermore, the threat of emerging resistance to available anti-*Pneumocystis* drugs highlights the need to continue to investigate the biology of this organism in the hope of developing novel treatment strategies.

References

[1] Revised nomenclature for Pneumocystis carinii. The *Pneumocystis* Workshop. *J Eukaryot Microbiol.* 1994; 41:S121-S122.

[2] Calderon-Sandubete EJ, Varela-Aguilar JM, Medrano-Ortega FJ, et al. Historical perspective on Pneumocystis *carinii* infection. *Protist* 2002;153:303-10.

[3] Van der Meer G, Brug SL. Infection a Pneumocystis chez l`homme et chez les animaux. *Ann Soc Belg Med Trop.* 1942; 22:301-7.

[4] Morris A, Lundgren JD, Masur H, et al. Current epidemiology of Pneumocystis Pneumonia. *Emerg Infect Dis.* 2004 ; 10 :1713-20.

[5] Hughes WT. Pneumocystis Pneumonitis in Non-HIV-Infected Patients: Update. In: *Pneumocystis carinii Pneumonia (3rd edition)*. Walzer PD, Cushion MT (eds.), Marcel Dekker, Inc., New York, 407-434 (2004).

[6] Peterson JC, Cushion MT. Pneumocystis: not just pneumonia. *Curr Opin Microbiol.* 2005; 8:393-8.

[7] Kaplan JE, Hanson D, Dworkin MS, et al. Epidemiology of human immunodeficiency virus-associated opportunistic infections in the United States in the era of highly active antiretroviral therapy. *Clin Infect Dis.* 2000; 30 (Suppl 1):S5-14.

[8] Magne D, Angoulvant A, Botterel F, et al. Réseau pneumocystose francilien : bilan de cinq années de surveillance (2003-2007). *J Mycol Med.* 2009;19:290-3.

[9] Calderón EJ, Varela JM, Medrano FJ, et al. Epidemiology of Pneumocystis carinii pneumonia in southern Spain. *Clin Microbiol Infect.* 2004; 10:673-6.

[10] Roblot F. Management of Pneumocystis pneumonia in patients with inflammatory disorders. *Expert Rev Anti Infect. Ther.* 2005; 3:435-44.

[11] Rodriguez M, Fishman JA. Prevention of infection due to Pneumocystis spp. in human immunodeficiency virus-negative immunocompromised patients. *Clin Microbiol Rev.* 2004; 17:770-82.

[12] Cardenal R, Medrano FJ, Varela JM, et al. Pneumocystis carinii pneumonia in heart transplant recipients. *Eur J Cardiothorac Surg.* 2001; 20:799-802.

[13] Takeuchi T, Tatsuki Y, Nogami Y, et al. Postmarketing surveillance of the safety profile of infliximab in 5000 Japanese patients with rheumatoid arthritis. *Ann Rheum Dis.* 2008; 67:189-94.
[14] Kalyoncu U, Karadag O, Akdogan A, et al. Pneumocystis carinii pneumonia in a rheumatoid arthritis patient treated with adalimumab. *Scand J Infect Dis.* 2007, 39:475-8.
[15] Lahiff C, Khiaron OB, Nolan N, Chadwick GA. *Pneumocystis carinii* pneumonia in a patient on etanercept for psoriatic arthritis. *Ir J Med Sci.* 2007; 176:309-11.
[16] Shelton E, Yong M, Cohney S. Late onset Pneumocystis pneumonia in patients receiving rituximab for humoral renal transplant rejection. *Nephrology* (Carlton). 2009; 14:696-9.
[17] Cruciani M, Marcati P, Malena M, Bosco O, Serpelloni G, Mengoli C. Meta-analysis of diagnostic procedures for Pneumocystis carinii pneumonia in HIV-1-infected patients. *Eur Respir. J.* 2002; 20:982-9.
[18] Thomas CF, Limper AH. Pneumocystis pneumonia. *N Engl J Med.* 2004; 350:2487-98.
[19] Aliouat-Denis CM, Martinez A, Aliouat el M, Pottier M, Gantois N, Dei-Cas E. The Pneumocystis life cycle. *Mem Inst Oswaldo Cruz.* 2009 ;104:419-26.
[20] Wazir JF, Ansari NA. Pneumocystis carinii infection. Update and review. *Arch Pathol Lab Med.* 2004; 128:1023-7.
[21] Krajicek BJ, Limper AH, Thomas CF. Advances in the biology, pathogenesis and identification of Pneumocystis pneumonia. *Curr Opin Pulm Med.* 2008; 14:228-34.
[22] Sepkowitz KA, Telzak EE, Gold JW, et al. Pneumothorax in AIDS. *Ann Intern Med.* 1991; 114:455-9.
[23] Krajicek BJ, Thomas CF, Limper AH. Pneumocystis pneumonia: current concepts in pathogenesis, diagnosis, and treatment. *Clin Chest Med.* 2009; 30:265-78.
[24] Kovacs JA, Masur H. Evolving health effects of Pneumocystis. *JAMA* 2009; 301:2578-85.
[25] Pyrgos V, Shoham S, Roilides E, Walsh TJ. Pneumocystis pneumonia in children. *Paediatr Respir Rev.* 2009; 10:192-8.
[26] Schliep TC, Yarrish RL. Pneumocystis carinii pneumonia. *Semin Respir Infect.* 1999; 14: 333-43.
[27] Nyamande K, Lalloo UG, Vawda F. Comparison of plain chest radiography and high-resolution CT in human immunodeficiency virus infected patients with community-acquired pneumonia: a sub-Saharan Africa study. *Br J Radiol.* 2007; 80:302-6.
[28] Mori S, Polatino S, Estrada-Y-Martin RM. Pneumocystis-associated organizing pneumonia as a manifestation of immune reconstitution inflammatory syndrome in an HIV-infected individual with a normal CD4+ T-cell count following antiretroviral therapy. *Int J STD AIDS* 2009; 20:662-5.
[29] Jagannathan P, Davis E, Jacobson M, Huang L. Life-threatening immune reconstitution inflammatory syndrome after Pneumocystis pneumonia: a cautionary case series. *AIDS* 2009; 23:1794-6.
[30] Cheng VC, Hung IF, Wu AK, Tang BS, Chu CM, Yuen KY. Lymphocyte surge as a marker for immunorestitution disease due to Pneumocystis jiroveci pneumonia in HIV-negative immunosuppressed hosts. *Eur J Clin Microbiol Infect Dis.* 2004; 23:512-4.

[31] Wislez M, Bergot E, Antoine M, et al. Acute respiratory failure following HAART introduction in patients treated for Pneumocystis carinii pneumonia. *Am J Respir Crit Care Med.* 2001; 164:847-51.

[32] Wu AK, Cheng VC, Tang BS, et al. The unmasking of Pneumocystis jiroveci pneumonia during reversal of immunosuppression: case reports and literature review. *BMC Infect Dis.* 2004; 4:57.

[33] Slivka A, Wen PY, Shea WM, Loeffler JS. Pneumocystis carinii pneumonia during steroid taper in patients with primary brain tumors. *Am J Med.* 1993; 94:216-9.

[34] Fulkerson WJ, Newman JH. Endogenous Cushing's syndrome complicated by Pneumocystis carinii pneumonia. *Am Rev Respir Dis.* 1984; 129:88-9.

[35] Ng VL, Yajko DM, Hadley WK. Extrapulmonary pneumocystosis. *Clin Microbiol Rev.* 1997; 10:401-18.

[36] Chalvardjian AM, Grawe LA. A new procedure for the identification of Pneumocystis carinii cysts in tissue sections and smears. *J Clin Pathol.* 1963; 16:383-4.

[37] Grocott RG. A stain for fungi in tissue sections and smears using Gomori's methenamine-silver nitrate technic. *Am J Clin Pathol.* 1955; 25:975-9.

[38] Walzer PD, Kim CK, Cushion MT. Pneumocystis carinii. In: *Parasitic Infections in the Compromised Host.* Walzer PD, Genta RM (eds.), Marcel Dekker, New York, 83-78 (1989).

[39] Yoshikawa H, Yoshida Y. Localization of silver deposits on Pneumocystis carinii treated with Gomori's methenamine silver nitrate stain. *Zentralbl Bakteriol Mikrobiol Hyg. A.* 1987; 264:363-72.

[40] Cushion MT, Ruffolo JJ, Linke MJ, Walzer PD. Pneumocystis carinii: growth variables and estimates in the A549 and WI-38 VA13 human cell lines. *Exp Parasitol.* 1985; 60:43-54.

[41] Dei-Cas E, Fleurisse L, Aliouat EM *et al.* Morphological and ultrastructural methods for Pneumocystis. *FEMS Immunol. Med Microbiol.* 1998; 22:185-9.

[42] Durand-Joly I, Wakefield AE, Palmer RJ *et al.* Ultrastructural and molecular characterization of Pneumocystis carinii isolated from a rhesus monkey (*Macaca mulatta*). *Med Mycol.* 2000; 38:61-72.

[43] Chouaid C, Housset B, Lebeau B. Cost-analysis of four diagnostic strategies for Pneumocystis carinii pneumonia in HIV-infected subjects. *Eur Respir J.* 1995; 8:1554-8.

[44] Dei-Cas E, Aliouat EM, Cailliez JC. Pneumocystis Cellular Structure. In: *Pneumocystis carinii Pneumonia, 3rd edition*, Walzer PD, Cushion MT (eds.), Marcel Dekker, Inc., New York, 61-94 (2004).

[45] Dei-Cas E, Chabé M, Moukhlis R *et al.* Pneumocystis oryctolagi sp. nov., an uncultured fungus causing pneumonia in rabbits at weaning: review of current knowledge, and description of a new taxon on genotypic, phylogenetic and phenotypic bases. *FEMS Microbiol. Rev.* 2006; 30:853-71.

[46] Kovacs JA, Ng VL, Masur H *et al.* Diagnosis of Pneumocystis carinii pneumonia: improved detection in sputum with use of monoclonal antibodies. *N Engl J Med.* 1988; 318:589-93.

[47] Limawongpranee S, Wanachiwanawin D, Chokephaibulkit K, Onchrotchanakun J, Lertlaituan P, Wankhom S. Sensitive detection of Pneumocystis jirovecii DNA in

gastric wash using nested polymerase chain reaction. *Southeast Asian J Trop Med Public Health* 2007; 38: 892-6.

[48] Aderaye G, Woldeamanuel Y, Asrat D et al. Evaluation of Toluidine Blue O staining for the diagnosis of Pneumocystis jiroveci in expectorated sputum sample and bronchoalveolar lavage from HIV-infected patients in a tertiary care referral center in Ethiopia. *Infection* 2008; 36:237-43.

[49] Broaddus C, Dake MD, Stulbarg MS, *et al.* Bronchoalveolar lavage and transbronchial biopsy for the diagnosis of pulmonary infections in the acquired immunodeficiency syndrome. *Ann Intern Med.* 1985; 102:747–52.

[50] Huang L, Hecht FM, Stansell JD, Montanti R, Hadley WK, Hopewell PC. Suspected Pneumocystis carinii pneumonia with a negative induced sputum examination: is early bronchoscopy useful? *Am J Respir Crit Care Med.* 1995; 151:1866–71.

[51] Wakefield AE, Pixley FJ, Banerji S *et al.* Detection of Pneumocystis carinii with DNA amplification. *Lancet* 1990; 336:451–3.

[52] Olsson M, Elvin K, Löfdahl S, Linder E. Detection of *Pneumocystis carinii* DNA in sputum and bronchoalveolar lavage samples by polymerase chain reaction. *J Clin Microbiol.* 1993; 31:221-6.

[53] De la Horra C, Varela JM, Friaza V, et al. Comparison of single and touchdown PCR protocols for detecting Pneumocystis jirovecii DNA in paraffin-embedded lung tissue samples. *J. Eukaryot. Microbiol.* 2006; 53 (Suppl 1):98-9.

[54] Durand-Joly I, Chabé M, Soula F, Delhaes L, Camus D, Dei-Cas E. Molecular diagnosis of Pneumocystis pneumonia (PcP). *FEMS Immunol. Med Microbiol.* 2005; 45:405-10.

[55] Durand-Joly, I., Soula, F., Chabe, M *et al.* Longterm colonization with Pneumocystis jirovecii in hospital staffs: a challenge to prevent nosocomial pneumocystosis. *J Eukaryot Microbiol.* 2003; 50 (Suppl.):614–5.

[56] Azoulay E, Bergeron A, Chevret S, Bele N, Schlemmer B, Menotti J. Polymerase chain reaction for diagnosing Pneumocystis pneumonia in non-HIV immunocompromised patients with pulmonary infiltrates. *Chest* 2009; 135:655-61.

[57] Respaldiza N, Montes-Cano MA, Friaza V, et al. Usefulness of oropharyngeal washings for identifying Pneumocystis jirovecii carriers. *J Eukaryo Microbiol.* 2006; 53(Suppl 1):100-1.

[58] Medrano FJ, Montes-Cano M, Conde M, et al. Pneumocystis jirovecii in general population. *Emerg Infect Dis.* 2005; 11:245-50.

[59] Nevez G, Chabé M, Rabodonirina M *et al.* Nosocomial Pneumocystis jirovecii infections. *Parasite* 2008; 15:359-365.

[60] Tsolaki AG, Miller RF, Wakefield AE. Oropharyngeal samples for genotyping and monitoring response to treatment in AIDS patients with Pneumocystis carinii pneumonia. *J. Med. Microbiol.* 1999; 48:897-905.

[61] Tamburrini E, Mencarini P, Visconti E *et al.* Potential impact of Pneumocystis genetic diversity on the molecular detection of the parasite in human host. *FEMS Immunol. Med. Microbiol.* 1998; 22:37-49.

[62] Huggett JF, Taylor MS, Kocjan G *et al.* Development and evaluation of a real-time PCR assay for detection of Pneumocystis jirovecii DNA in bronchoalveolar lavage fluid of HIV-infected patients. *Thorax* 63, 154-159 (2008).

[63] Huang L. Clinical presentation and diagnosis of Pneumocystis pneumonia in HIV-infected patients. In: *Pneumocystis carinii Pneumonia, 3rd edition*, Walzer PD, Cushion MT (eds.), Marcel Dekker, Inc., New York, 349-406 (2004).
[64] Durand-Joly I. Épidémiologie moléculaire de la pneumocystose humaine. Caractérisation génétique et phénotypique de Pneumocystis jirovecii et espèces proches. *Thesis Dissertation* Lille (2002).
[65] Wakefield AE, Miller RF, Guiver LA, Hopkin JM. Oropharyngeal samples for detection of Pneumocystis carinii by DNA amplification. *Q J Med.* 1993; 86:401-6.
[66] Helweg-Larsen J, Jensen JS, Lundgren B. Noninvasive diagnosis of Pneumocystis carinii pneumonia in haematological patients using PCR on oral washes. *J Eukaryo. Microbiol.* 1997; 44 (Suppl):59.
[67] Khan MA, Farrag N, Butcher P. Diagnosis of Pneumocystis carinii pneumonia: immunofluorescence staining, simple PCR or nPCR. . *Infect.* 1999; 39:77–80.
[68] Richards CG, Wakefield AE, Mitchell CD. Detection of Pneumocystis DNA in nasopharyngeal aspirates of leukaemic infants with pneumonia. *Arch Dis Child.* 1994; 71: 254–5.
[69] Larsen HH, Huang L, Kovacs JA et al. A prospective, blinded study of quantitative touch-down polymerase chain reaction using oral-wash samples for diagnosis of Pneumocystis pneumonia in HIV-infected patients. *J Infect Dis.* 2004; 189:1679–83.
[70] Calderon EJ. Epidemiology of Pneumocystis infection in human. *J Mycol Med.*2009; 19: 270-5.
[71] Larsen HH, Masur H, Kovacs JA et al. Development and evaluation of a quantitative, touchdown, real-time PCR assay for diagnosing Pneumocystis carinii pneumonia. *J Clin Microbiol.* 2002; 40, 490–4.
[72] Morris A, Wei K, Afshar K, Huang L. Epidemiology and clinical significance of Pneumocystis colonization. *J Infect Dis.*12008; 97:10-17.
[73] Vidal S, de la Horra C, Martín J, et al. Pneumocystis jirovecii colonisation in patients with interstitial lung disease. *Clin Microbiol Infect.* 2006; 12 :231-5.
[74] Chabé M, Dei-Cas E, Creusy C et al. Immunocompetent hosts as a reservoir of Pneumocystis organisms: histological and RT-PCR data demonstrate active replication. *Eur J Clin Microbiol Infect Dis.* 2004; 23:89-97.
[75] Calderón EJ, Rivero L, Respaldiza N et al. Systemic inflammation in patients with chronic obstructive pulmonary disease who are colonized with Pneumocystis jirovecii. *Clin Infect Dis.* 2007; 45:17-19.
[76] Tan WC, Ng TP. COPD in Asia: where east meets west. *Chest* 2008; 133:517–27.
[77] Miller RF, Wakefield AE. *Pneumocystis carinii* genotypes and severity of pneumonia. *Lancet* 1999; 353:2039-40.
[78] Totet A, Pautard JC, Raccurt C, Roux P, Nevez G. Genotypes at the internal transcribed spacers of the nuclear rRNA operon of Pneumocystis jirovecii in nonimmunosuppressed infants without severe pneumonia. *J Clin Microbiol.* 2003; 41:1173-80.
[79] Beard CB. Molecular typing and epidemiological insights. In: *Pneumocystis carinii Pneumonia (3rd edition).* Walzer PD, Cushion MT (eds.), Marcel Dekker, Inc., New York, 479-504 (2004).

[80] Beser J, Hagblom P, Fernandez V. Frequent in vitro recombination in internal transcribed spacers 1 and 2 during genotyping of Pneumocystis jirovecii. *J Clin Microbiol*. 2007; 45:881-6.
[81] Friaza V, Montes-Cano MA, Respaldiza N, Morilla R, Calderón EJ, de la Horra C. Prevalence of dihydropteroate synthase mutations in Spanish patients with HIV-associated Pneumocystis pneumonia. *Diagn Microbiol Infect Dis*. 2009; 64:104-5.
[82] Iliades P, Meshnick SR, Macreadie IG. Dihydropteroate synthase mutations in Pneumocystis jiroveci can affect sulfamethoxazole resistance in a Saccharomyces cerevisiae model. *Antimicrob Agents Chemother*. 2004; 48;2617-23.
[83] Nahimana A, Rabodonirina M, Bille J, Francioli P, Hauser PM. Mutations of Pneumocystis jirovecii dihydrofolate reductase associated with failure of prophylaxis. *Antimicrob Agents Chemother*. 2004: 48:4301-5.
[84] Huang L, Crothers K, Atzori C et al. Dihydropteroate synthase gene mutations in Pneumocystis and sulfa resistance. *Emerg Infect Dis*. 2004; 10:1721–8.
[85] Kazanjian P, Armstrong W, Hossler PA *et al.* Pneumocystis carinii mutations are associated with duration of sulfa or sulfone prophylaxis exposure in AIDS patients. *J Infect Dis*. 2000; 182:551–7.
[86] Huang L, Beard CB, Creasman J *et al.* Sulfa or sulfone prophylaxis and geographic region predict mutations in the Pneumocystis carinii dihydropteroate synthase gene. *J Infect Dis*.2000; 182:1192–8.
[87] Helweg-Larsen J, Benfield TL, Eugen-Olsen J, Lundgren JD, Lundgren B. Effects of mutations in Pneumocystis carinii dihydropteroate synthase gene on outcome of AIDS-associated *P. carinii* pneumonia. *Lancet* 1999; 354:1347–51.
[88] Valerio A, Tronconi E, Mazza F *et al.* Genotyping *of Pneumocystis jirovecii* pneumonia in Italian AIDS patients. Clinical outcome is influenced by dihydropteroate synthase and not by internal transcribed spacer genotype. *J Acquir Immune Defic Syndr*. 2007; 45:521–8.
[89] Alvarez-Martínez MJ, Moreno A, Miró JM et al. Pneumocystis jirovecii pneumonia in Spanish HIV-infected patients in the combined antiretroviral therapy era: prevalence of dihydropteroate synthase mutations and prognostic factors of mortality. *Diagn Microbiol Infect Dis*. 2008; 62:34-43.
[90] van Hal SJ, Gilgado F, Doyle T *et al.* Clinical significance and phylogenetic relationship of novel Australian Pneumocystis jirovecii genotypes. *J Clin Microbiol*. 2009; 47:1818-23.
[91] Stein CR, Poole C, Kazanjian P, Meshnick SR. Sulfa use, Dihydropteroate sythase mutations, and Pneumocystis jirovecii pneumonia. *Emerg Infect Dis*.2004; 10:1760-5.
[92] Navin T R, Beard CB, Huang L *et al.* Effect of mutations in Pneumocystis carinii dihydropteroate synthase gene on outcome of P. carinii pneumonia in patients with HIV-1: a prospective study. *Lancet* 2001; 358: 545–9.
[93] Calderon E, de la Horra C, Montes-Cano MA, Respaldiza N, Martín-Juan J, Varela JM. Resistencia genotípica a sulfamidas en pacientes con neumonía por Pneumocystis jiroveci. *Med. Clin. (Barc) 2004;* 122:617-9.
[94] Thomas CF Jr, Limper AH. Current insights into the biology and pathogenesis of Pneumocystis pneumonia. *Nat Rev Microbiol*. 2007; 5:298-308.
[95] Desmet S, Van Wijngaerden E, Maertens J *et al.* Serum (1-3)-beta-D-glucan as a tool for diagnosis of Pneumocystis jirovecii pneumonia in patients with human

immunodeficiency virus infection or hematological malignancy. *J Clin Microbiol.* 2009; 47:3871-4.

[96] Teramoto S, Sawaki D, Okada S, Ouchi Y. Markedly increased plasma (1-->3)-beta-D-glucan is a diagnostic and therapeutic indicator of Pneumocystis carinii pneumonia in a non-AIDS patient. *J Med Microbiol.* 2000; 49:393-4.

[97] Nakamura H, Tateyama M, Tasato D *et al.* Clinical utility of serum beta-D-glucan and KL-6 levels in Pneumocystis jirovecii pneumonia. *Intern Med.* 2009; 48:195-202.

[98] Tasaka S, Hasegawa N, Kobayashi S, et al. Serum indicators for the diagnosis of pneumocystis pneumonia. *Chest.* 2007;131:1173-80.

[99] Pontón J. Utilidad de los marcadores biológicos en el diagnóstico de la candidiasis invasora. *Rev Iberoam Micol.* 2009; 26:8-14.

[100] Clarkson AB, Merali S. Polyamines, Iron, and Pneumocystis carinii. In: *Pneumocystis carinii Pneumonia (3rd edition)*, Walzer PD, Cushion MT (eds.), Marcel Dekker, Inc., New York, 577-605 (2004).

[101] Skelly M, Hoffman J, Fabbri M, Holzman RS, Clarkson AB Jr, Merali S. S-adenosylmethionine concentrations in diagnosis of Pneumocystis carinii pneumonia. *Lancet* 2003; 361:1267–8.

[102] Skelly MJ, Holzman RS, Merali S. S-adenosylmethionine levels in the diagnosis of Pneumocystis carinii pneumonia in patients with HIV infection. *Clin Infect Dis.* 2008; 46:467–71.

[103] Wang P, Huang L, Davis JL et al. A hydrophilic-interaction chromatography tandem mass spectrometry method for quantitation of serum s-adenosylmethionine in patients infected with human immunodeficiency virus. *Clin Chim Acta* 2008; 396:86-8.

[104] Kutty G, Hernandez-Novoa B, Czapiga M, Kovacs JA. Pneumocystis encodes a functional S-adenosylmethionine synthetase gene. *Eukaryot Cell* 2008; 7:258–67.

[105] Sato H, Callister ME, Mumby S, et al. KL-6 levels are elevated in plasma from patients with acute respiratory distress syndrome. *Eur Respir J.* 2004; 23:142-5.

[106] Inoue Y, Nishimura K, Shiode M, et al. Evaluation of serum KL-6 levels in patients with pulmonary tuberculosis. *Tuber Lung Dis.* 1995; 76:230-3.

[107] Sukoh N, Yamamoto H, Kikuchi E, et al. A case of severe Legionella pneumonia monitored with serum SP-A, SP-D, and KL-6. *Nihon Kokyuki Gakkai Zasshi.* 2001; 39:126-30.

[108] Kawasaki Y, Aoyagi Y, Abe Y, et al. Serum KL-6 levels as a biomarker of lung injury in respiratory syncytial virus bronchiolitis. *J Med Virol.* 2009; 81:2104-8.

[109] Walzer PD. Immunological Features of *Pneumocystis* Infection in Humans. In: *Pneumocystis carinii Pneumonia, 3rd edition*, Walzer PD, Cushion MT (eds.), Marcel Dekker, Inc., New York, 451-477 (2004).

[110] Daly K, Koch J, Respaldiza N *et al.* Geographical variation in serological responses to recombinant Pneumocystis jirovecii major surface glycoprotein antigens. *Clin Microbiol Infect.* 2009; 15:937-42.

[111] Miller RF, Le Noury J, Corbett EL, Felton JM, De Cock KM. Pneumocystis carinii infection: current treatment and prevention. *J Antimicrob Chemother.* 1996; 37 (Suppl B):33-53.

[112] Centers for Disease Control and Prevention. Guidelines for Prevention and Treatment of Opportunistic Infections in HIV-Infected Adults and Adolescents. *MMWR* 2009; 58:1-216.

[113] Larsen HH, Masur H, Kovacs JA. Current regimens for treatment and prophylaxis of Pneumocystis jiroveci pneumonia. In: *Pneumocystis carinii Pneumonia, 3rd edition*, Walzer PD, Cushion MT (eds.), Marcel Dekker, Inc., New York, 505-538 (2004).
[114] Smego RA Jr, Nagar S, Maloba B, Popara M. A meta-analysis of salvage therapy for *Pneumocystis carinii* pneumonia. *Arch Intern Med.* 2001; 161:1529-33.
[115] Benfield T, Atzori C, Miller RF, Helweg-Larsen J. Second-line salvage treatment of AIDS-associated Pneumocystis jirovecii pneumonia: a case series and systematic review. *J Acquir Immune Defic Syndr.* 2008; 48:63-7.
[116] Zolopa A, Andersen J, Powderly W, et al. Early antiretroviral therapy reduces AIDS progression/death in individuals with acute opportunistic infections: a multicenter randomized strategy trial. *PLoS One* 2009; 4, e5575.
[117] Helweg-Larsen J, Benfield T, Atzori C, Miller RF. Clinical efficacy of first- and second-line treatments for HIV-associated Pneumocystis jirovecii pneumonia: a tri-centre cohort study. *J Antimicrob Chemother.* 2009; 64:1282-90.
[118] Mofenson LM, Brady MT, Danner SP, et al. Guidelines for the Prevention and Treatment of Opportunistic Infections among HIV-exposed and HIV-infected children: recommendations from CDC, the National Institutes of Health, the HIV Medicine Association of the Infectious Diseases Society of America, the Pediatric Infectious Diseases Society, and the American Academy of Pediatrics. *MMWR Recomm Rep.* 2009; 58 (RR-11):1-166.
[119] Crothers K, Beard CB, Turner J, et al. Severity and outcome of HIV-associated *Pneumocystis* pneumonia containing Pneumocystis jirovecii dihydropteroate synthase gene mutations. *AIDS* 2005; 19:801-5.
[120] Eeftinck Schattenkerk JK, Lange JM, van Steenwijk RP, Danner SA. Can the course of high dose cotrimoxazole for Pneumocystis carinii pneumonia in AIDS be shorter? A possible solution to the problem of cotrimoxazole toxicity. *J Intern Med.* 1990; 227:359-62.
[121] Gordin FM, Simon GL, Wofsy CB, Mills J. Adverse reactions to trimethoprim-sulfamethoxazole in patients with the acquired immunodeficiency syndrome. *Ann Intern Med.* 1984; 100:495-9.
[122] Hughes WT, LaFon SW, Scott JD, Masur H. Adverse events associ¬ated with trimethoprim-sulfamethoxazole and atovaquone during the treatment of AIDS-related Pneumocystis carinii pneumonia. *J Infect Dis.* 1995; 171:1295-1301.
[123] Conte JE, Jr., Chernoff D, Feigal DW, Jr., et al. Intravenous or inhaled pentamidine for treating Pneumocystis carinii pneumonia in AIDS: a randomized trial. *Ann Intern Med.* 1990; 113:203-9.
[124] O'Brien JG, Dong BJ, Coleman RL, Gee L, Balano KB. A 5-year retrospective review of adverse drug reactions and their risk factors in HIV-infected patients who were receiving intravenous therapy for Pneumocystis carinii pneumonia. *Clin Infect Dis.* 1997; 24:854-9.
[125] Black JR, Feinberg J, Murphy RL, Fass RJ, Finkelstein D, and Akil B. Clindamycin and primaquine therapy for mild-to-moderate episodes of Pneumocystis carinii pneumonia in patients with AIDS (ACTG 044). *Clin Infect Dis.* 1994; 18:905-13.
[126] Toma E, Thorne A, Singer J, et al. Clindamycin with primaquine vs. Trimethoprim-sulfamethoxazole therapy for mild and moderately severe Pneumocystis carinii

pneumonia in patients with AIDS: a multicenter, double-blind, randomized trial. *Clin Infect Dis.* 1998; 27, 524-30.

[127] Medina I, Mills J, Leoung G, et al. Oral therapy for Pneumocystis carinii pneumonia in the acquired immunodeficiency syndrome: a controlled trial of trimethoprim–sulfamethoxazole versus trimethoprim-dapsone. *N. Engl. J. Med.* 323, 776-782 (1990).

[128] Baggish AL, Hill DR. Antiparasitic agent atovaquone. *Antimicrob Agents Chemother.* 2002; 46:1163-73.

[129] Kazanjian P, Armstrong W, Hossler P.A, et al. Pneumocystis carinii cytochrome b mutations are associated with atovaquone exposure in patients with AIDS. *J Infect Dis* 2001; 183:819-22.

[130] Kovacs JA, Allegra CJ, Kennedy S, et al. Efficacy of trimetrexate, a potent lipid-soluble antifolate, in the treatment of rodent Pneumocystis carinii pneumonia. *Am J Trop Med Hyg.* 1988; 39:491-6.

[131] Allegra CJ., Kovacs JA, Drake JC, Swan JC, Chabner BA. and Masur H. Activity of antifolates against Pneumocystis carinii dihydrofolate reductase and identification of a potent new agent. *J Exp Med.* 1987; 165:926-31.

[132] Sattler FR, Frame P, Davis R, et al. Trimetrexate with leucovorin versus trimethoprim-sulfamethoxazole for moderate to severe episodes of *Pneumocystis carinii* pneumonia in patients with AIDS: a prospective, controlled multicenter investigation of the AIDS Clinical Trials Group Protocol 029/031. *J Infect Dis.* 1994; 170:165-72.

[133] Short CE, Gilleece YC, Fisher MJ, Churchill DR. Trimetrexate and folinic acid: a valuable salvage option for Pneumocystis jirovecii pneumonia. *AIDS* 2009; 23:1287-90.

[134] Briel M, Boscacci R, Furrer H, Bucher HC. Adjunctive corticosteroids for Pneumocystis jiroveci pneumonia in patients with HIV infection: a meta-analysis of randomised controlled trials. *BMC Infect Dis.* 2005; 5:101.

[135] Pareja JG, Garland R, Koziel H. Use of adjunctive corticosteroids in severe adult non-HIV *Pneumocystis carinii* pneumonia. *Chest* 1998; 113:1215-4.

[136] Herreros E, Martinez CM, Almela MJ, Marriott MS, De Las Heras FG, Gargallo-Viola D. Sordarins: in vitro activities of new antifungal derivatives against pathogenic yeasts, Pneumocystis carinii, and filamentous fungi. *Antimicrob. Agents Chemother.* 1998; 42:2863-9.

[137] Aviles P, Aliouat EM, Martinez A, et al. In vitro pharmacodynamic parameters of sordarin derivatives in comparison with those of marketed compounds against *Pneumocystis carinii* isolated from rats. *Antimicrob Agents Chemother*. 2000; 44:1284-90.

[138] Powles MA, Liberator P, Anderson J, et al. Efficacy of MK-991 (L- 743,872), a semisynthetic Pneumocandin, in murine models of Pneumocystis carinii. *Antimicrob Agents Chemother.* 1998; 42:1985-9.

[139] Utili R, Durante-Mangoni E, Basilico C, Mattei A, Ragone E, Grossi P. Efficacy of caspofungin addition to trimethoprim-sulfamethoxazole treatment for severe Pneumocystis pneumonia in solid organ transplant recipients. *Transplantation* 2007; 84:685-8.

[140] Xiang-dong MU, Cheng-li QUE, Bing HE, Wang Guang-fa, Hai-chao LI. Caspofungin in salvage treatment of severe *Pneumocystis* pneumonia: case report and literature review. *Chin Med J. (Engl)* 2009; 122:996-9.

[141] Fei MW, Kim EJ, Sant CA, et al. Predicting mortality from HIV-associated *Pneumocystis* pneumonia at illness presentation: an observational cohort study. *Thorax*. 2009; 64:1070-6.

[142] Catherinot E, Lanternier F, Bougnoux ME, Lecuit M, Couderc LJ, Lortholary O. Pneumocystis jirovecii Pneumonia. *Infect Dis Clin North Am*. 2010; 24:07-38.

[143] Green H, Paul M, Vidal L, Leibovici L. Prophylaxis of Pneumocystis pneumonia in immunocompromised non-HIV-infected patients: systematic review and meta-analysis of randomized controlled trials. *Mayo Clin Proc*. 2007; 82:1052-9.

[144] Di Cocco P, Orlando G, Bonanni L, et al. A systematic review of two different trimetoprim-sulfamethoxazole regimens used to prevent Pneumocystis jirovecii and no prophylaxis at all in transplant recipients: appraising the evidence. *Transplant Proc*. 2009; 41: 1201-3.

[145] Podzamczer D, Salazar A, Jimenez J, et al. Intermittent trimethoprim-sulfamethoxazole compared with dapsone-pyrimethamine for the simultaneous primary prophylaxis of Pneumocystis pneumonia and toxoplasmosis in patients infected with HIV. *Ann Intern Med*. 1995; 122:755–61.

[146] El-Sadr WM, Murphy RL, Yurik TM, et al. Atovaquone compared with dapsone for the prevention of *Pneumocystis carinii* pneumonia in patients with HIV infection who cannot tolerate trimethoprim, sulfonamides, or both. *N Engl J Med*. 1998; 339:1889–95.

[147] Huang L, Morris A, Limper AH, Beck JM; ATS Pneumocystis Workshop Participants. An Official ATS Workshop Summary: Recent advances and future directions in *Pneumocystis* pneumonia (PCP). *Proc Am Thorac Soc*. 2006; 3:655-64.

[148] Yale SH, Limper AH. *Pneumocystis carinii* pneumonia in patients without acquired immunodeficiency syndrome: associated illness and prior corticosteroid therapy. *Mayo Clin. Proc*. 1996; 71:5-13.

[149] Sowden E, Carmichael AJ. Autoimmune inflammatory disorders, systemic corticosteroids and *Pneumocystis* pneumonia: a strategy for prevention. *BMC Infect Dis*. 2004; 4:42.

[150] Lemaire CM, Browning JC, Hsu S. Medical pearl: *Pneumocystis* pneumonia prophylaxis for patients on chronic systemic corticosteroids. *J Am Acad Dermatol*. 2006; 55:24-5.

[151] Langford CA, Talar-Williams C, Barron KS, Sneller MC. Use of cyclophosphamide-induction methotrexate-maintenance regimen for the treatment of Wegener's granulomatosis: extended follow-up and rate of relapse. *Am J Med*. 2003; 114:463–9.

[152] Wegener's Granulomatosis Etanercept Trial (WGET) Research Group. Etanercept plus standard therapy for Wegener's granulomatosis. *N Engl J Med*. 2005; 352:351-61.

[153] Lopez Bernaldo de Quiros JC, Miro JM, Peña JM, et al. A randomized trial of the discontinuation of primary and secondary prophylaxis against Pneumocystis carinii pneumonia after highly active antiretroviral therapy in patients with HIV infection. *N Engl J Med*. 2001; 344:159-67.

In: Pneumonia: Symptoms, Diagnosis and Treatment
Editors: M. L. Suarez and S. M. Ortega, pp. 37-62
ISBN: 978-1-61209-685-8

Chapter II

Supportive Treatment to Improve Outcome of Pneumonia

Michael Eisenhut and Tomasz Rajkowski
Paediatric Department, Luton&Dunstable Hospital NHS Foundation Trust, Lewsey Road
Luton, LU4ODZ, United Kingdom

Abstract

Pneumonia is one of the most common serious infections, causing two million deaths annually among young children in low-income countries. It is the largest killer, accounting for 28 to 34% of all child deaths below five years of age in low income countries and is an important cause of mortality in the elderly in high-income countries. Despite availability of effective antibiotic treatment the mortality remains 6 to 12% in patients admitted to hospital with community acquired pneumonia and over 50% in patients admitted to the intensive care unit (figures from the United Kingdom). The objective of this review is to summarize evidence for the effectiveness of modes of supportive treatment in patients with pneumonia. Supportive treatment explored in patients with pneumonia includes oxygen in a variety of applications, fluid therapy regimens, chest physiotherapy, steroid treatment, granulocyte colony stimulating factor treatment, surfactant application and vitamins A, C and D, zinc, protein and calorie supplements. Studies showed that management of patients with monitoring of oxygen levels and oxygen delivery guided by oxygen saturation levels can reduce hospitalisation. In children four randomised controlled trials compared oxygen delivery methods and found that nasal prongs and nasopharyngeal catheters were found to be similar in effectiveness and safety. Review of trials, which assessed the accuracy of clinical signs indicating hypoxemia found that no single clinical sign or symptom accurately identified hypoxemia. Vitamin C supplementation in critically ill patients was associated with lower mortality and reduced respiratory symptom score in one trial. Steroid application was associated with reduction of mortality and need for mechanical ventilation in people with pneumocystis jiroveci pneumonia but there has been insufficient evidence supporting their use in other forms of pneumonia. Use of granulocyte colony stimulating factor application was not associated with reduction of mortality in a meta-analysis of 6 studies. Six trials investigating vitamin A showed no significant reduction in mortality or duration of hospital stay but demonstrated a 39% reduction in antibiotic first line failure (OR 0.65: 95% CI 0.42 to 1.01). Trials using supplementation with zinc did not show consistent benefit. For fluid regimes, chest physiotherapy, vitamin D and protein and calorie supplements there has been a lack of evidence for an influence on outcome and further research is required.

1. Introduction

Pneumonia is one of the most common serious infections, causing two million deaths annually among young children in low-income countries. It is the largest killer, accounting for 28 to 34% of all child deaths below five years of age in low-income countries and is an important cause of mortality in the elderly in high-income countries. Despite availability of effective antibiotic treatment the mortality remains 6 to 12% in patients admitted to hospital with community-acquired pneumonia and over 50% in patients admitted to the intensive care unit (figures from the United Kingdom). The objective of this review is to summarize evidence for the effectiveness of modes of supportive treatment in patients with pneumonia, which as an adjunct to antibiotic therapy could improve outcome. Included in the review were all modes of supportive treatment like oxygen therapy, physiotherapy, medication, fluid therapy, micronutrients and nutritional supplements. Emphasis was placed on presentation of high quality evidence from randomized controlled trials. Negative as well as positive findings are presented. Databases searched included MEDLINE and PUBMED and the Cochrane Library. To understand the rationale of use of supportive treatment research explaining the mechanisms of effect of the investigated interventions is also described.

2. Oxygen Therapy

2.1. Historical Background of Therapeutic use of Oxygen in Medicine

The first published case of oxygen use as a remedy took place in 1783 and was described by the French physician Caillens (Smith 1870). Since than according to Professor Martin:

> "Although oxygen's life-supporting role was understood early on, it took about 150 years for the gas to be used in a proper fashion for patients. For the first 150 years after discovery, therapeutic use of oxygen was sporadic, erratic, controversial, comical, beset by quackery, and only occasionally helpful" (Martin 1998).

It was not until the beginnings of the 20th century when due to works of Haldane, Barcroft and others, oxygen therapy was placed on a rational, scientific basis. Interestingly in the first two decades of the 20th century there were numerous papers about intra-abdominal, intravenous, rectal, and subcutaneous administration of oxygen with some case reports mentioning therapeutic success of these interventions (Martin 1998). The modern era of oxygen therapy began after World War I. In 1917 Haldane published his work about an addition of oxygen to the inspired air (from oxygen cylinders) via facial mask to persons intoxicated with toxic war gases. He described many physiological details and was also aware of possible side effects of providing pure oxygen inhalations (Haldane 1917). Haldane pointed out that, because the body does not have any stores of oxygen, if there is a need, oxygen must be delivered continuously. He also developed equipment for a cheap and efficient way of providing oxygen to patients. The same year Meltzer published a paper discussing the therapeutic value of oxygen delivered under positive pressure (Meltzer 1917). Subsequent works of Haldane, Barcroft and others at that time gave scientific background to the physiological role of oxygen and its therapeutic use in current medicine.

2.2. History of Oxygen use in Pneumonia

The first report about use of oxygen in patients suffering with pneumonia was published in 1887. In this case report Holtzapple described a 16 year old patient with high fever, productive cough, tachypnoea (> 75 breaths/minute!) and cyanosis who fully recovered after intermitted use of oxygen for just 1 day (Shultz 2005).

The first experimental data about use of oxygen in animals with laboratory evoked pneumonia were published by Binger in 1928. He injected streptococci directly into lungs of anesthetized guinea pigs and then kept some of them in atmospheric air and others in 50% of oxygen. He noticed that 66 of 70 (94%) guinea pigs kept in air died within 2 weeks compared with only 22 of 45 (49%) of those kept in enriched oxygen atmosphere. This was the first experimental observation suggesting a beneficial role of oxygen therapy in decreasing mortality in pneumonia. (Binger 1928).

In 1919 Stadie published a review of 33 patients with pneumonia in whom he measured oxygen content in venous and arterial blood and described a connection between low concentration of oxygen in the blood and cyanosis. In summary he wrote:

> "It is evident that the cyanosis of pneumonia patients is due to the incomplete saturation of venous blood with oxygen in the lungs, and that the various shades of blue observed in the distal parts are caused by an admixture of reduced hemoglobin and oxyhemoglobin in the superficial capillaries (Stadie 1919).

Results from this paper and other retrospective studies from the twenties of the XX century were clearly suggesting a connection between mortality from pneumonia in humans with low oxygen saturation of the arterial blood, presence of bacteraemia, the serotype of the organism and the age of patient (WHO 1993). In this pre antibiotic era, mortality adjusted to the severity of illness was 39% with oxygen use and 74% without oxygen therapy (table 1 from WHO 1993).

In 1927 Prendergast compared medical use and costs of nasal tubes, Haldane masks and oxygen chambers as different methods of oxygen administration to pneumonia sufferers and suggested that nasal tube "is perhaps the best of them for general use" (Prendergast 1927). In this paper he mentioned that, although he did not have exact data of the effect of oxygen on mortality in pneumonia, starting the treatment early before cyanosis develops should be considered as a logical option.

During the 2nd World War a new era of pneumonia treatment started with the discovery of penicillin. In subsequent years more controlled, safe and cheaper oxygen cylinders and oxygen concentrators were developed enabling wider use of oxygen in medicine. At the same time delivery methods of oxygen, other that through inhalation, were abandoned. Below we present a review of the current evidence for use of oxygen in patients with pneumonia. The majority of available data are from studies in the paediatric population.

Table 1 Effect of oxygen therapy on mortality from pneumonia (from WHO 1993)

	Died /total (% died)	
	Without oxygen	With oxygen
Saturation* <80% and bacteraemia	2/2/(100)	15/21 (71)
Saturation <80% and no bacteraemia	12/13 (92)	19/52 (37)
Saturation ≥80% and bacteraemia	2/4 (50)	3/8 (38)
Saturation ≥80% and no bacteraemia	2/15 (13)	1/12 (17)
Total, adjusted for severity of illness	74 % died	39% died

*Saturation represents oxygen saturation of arterial blood

2.3. Hypoxia and Mortality

Hypoxemia is a major complication and cause of deterioration in pneumonia and is associated with a significantly increased mortality risk (Theodoratou 2010). Both the severity of pneumonia and hypoxia correlate strongly with mortality (WHO 2007). A systematic review of cohort studies reporting the frequency of hypoxemia in 4,021 children less than 5 years of age with acute lower respiratory infections showed a prevalence of hypoxemia of 43% in patients with clinical pneumonia and 72% in those with radiographically confirmed pneumonia (Lozano 2001). An association between hypoxemia and death was reported there with relative risks varying between 1.4 and 4.6. The author concluded that in view of above findings efforts should be made to improve the detection of hypoxemia and to provide oxygen earlier to more children with severe acute lower respiratory tract infections. Even more striking results come from another prospective cohort study in Gambia (Usen 1999). Amongst 1072 children, aged 2 to 33 months, who were admitted with an acute lower respiratory tract infection to hospitals 63 (5.9%) were hypoxemic (having an arterial oxygen saturation <90%). Children with hypoxemia were five times more likely to die than non-hypoxemic children. Mentioned previously, a recent systematic review of the literature with the aim to assess the effect of pneumonia case management on mortality from childhood pneumonia (Theodoratou 2010) identified one study demonstrating the effectiveness of oxygen therapy on decrease of mortality in pneumonia (Duke 2008). In that multi-hospital study from Papua New Guinea authors compared mortality before and after implementation of an improved oxygen system in hospitals (oxygen concentrators and pulsoximetry measurement). They observed reduction in mortality from 4.9 to 3.2% (decrease by 35%), and the overall mortality risk was significantly reduced by the improved system (risk ratio 0.65, p<0,0001). Apart from the new oxygen system there was no other change in management of sick children so decrease in mortality may be attributed only to improved oxygen therapy.

2.4. Studies Comparing use of Oxygen Versus no Oxygen Therapy

A Cochrane review of 551 medical titles (1966 to 2008) about oxygen therapy in children (Royas-Reyes 2009) was not able to identify any studies comparing oxygen versus no oxygen therapy in lower respiratory tract infections. This is because any study in which some hypoxic patients are deprived of oxygen therapy would be considered unethical (Dyke 1994).

2.5. Indications for Oxygen Therapy in Pneumonia

The World Health Organization recommends oxygen treatment in pneumonia if oxygen saturation is below 90% (WHO 2005) or, if pulse oximetry is not available, oxygen should be used for children with severe pneumonia presenting with cyanosis or inability to feed (WHO 1993). Hypoxemia is a generally accepted indication for oxygen therapy in pneumonia (WHO 1993, WHO 2005, BTS 2002, BTS 2008, BTS 2009). Hypoxemia is defined as lower than normal value of partial pressure of oxygen in the blood (PaO2) assessed by invasive blood gas analysis or as an arterial oxygen saturation (SaO2) decreased below norm as assessed by pulse oximetry. The latter, due to its simplicity and non invasive character, is used as a gold standard in assessment of hypoxemia (Royas-Reyes 2009, Duke 2008). Unfortunately there is no universally agreed lower limit of normal oxygen saturation (Royas-Reyes 2009). In 12 observational studies included for review by Royas the cut off value for diagnosis of hypoxemia was between 82 and 93% on different altitudes above sea level (3750 and 35 masl respectively) (Royas-Reyes 2009). The cut off values therefore had to be determined by studying healthy children from the same population. This physiological decrease in SaO2 with increasing altitude above sea level makes comparison between studies from different countries more difficult. Moreover in low income countries where health resources are limited pulse oximeters may not be available. Therefore health workers have to determine presence of hypoxemia (as an indicator for hospitalization and oxygen therapy) based on clinical signs and symptoms.

2.6. Clinical Indicators of Hypoxemia

Clinical signs frequently mentioned as indicators of hypoxemia are: cyanosis, grunting, nasal flaring, tachypnoea, chest indrawing, crepitations, restlessness and inability to drink (WHO 1993, Royas-Reyes 2009, Ayeko 2006, Dyke 1994).

The first available analysis of clinical criteria related to hypoxia in children with pneumonia was presented in the document prepared by the Programme for the Control of Acute Respiratory Infections of the World Health Organization (WHO 1993). After review of the contemporary literature authors of the report concluded that from all considered signs only central cyanosis is strongly related to both hypoxemia and mortality in pneumonia.

Interestingly authors quoted observation from a Kenyan study (Onyango 1993) where mother's perception of cyanosis was the best single predictor of hypoxemia in infants below 3 months of age. Inability to drink was assessed as "related" to mortality and in view of little data relationship to hypoxemia was not assessed. Other considered parameters (severe chest indrawing, respiratory rate > 70 breaths per minute, grunting in infants below 2 months of age and restlessness) were found to be not or only weekly related to hypoxemia and mortality in pneumonia. As methodology leading to these conclusions is not presented in this paper it is not possible to critically review these data.

Royas-Reyes with collaborators, after systematic review of the literature, extracted 12 observational studies assessing the accuracy of clinical signs indicating hypoxemia (Royas-Reyes 2009). In view of heterogeneity in the population baseline characteristics between studies meta-analysis was not performed. Authors combined results showing sensitivity and specificity for each sign (see summary in table 2) compared with oxygen saturation results. Similar to the WHO document, this review confirmed that cyanosis is a very specific sign in determining the presence of hypoxemia (specificity 75-100%) but sensitivity was very variable between studies and not related to age group or the altitude. Similar results were found for the inability to drink/feed (specificity 60 –99 with variable sensitivity 28-71%). According to WHO recommendations (WHO 1993) inability to drink is the second clinical sign (apart from cyanosis) which, when present in child with pneumonia, should prompt health professional to commence oxygen therapy. Specificity for grunting and alteration in mental status were good indicators and consistent between studies but again sensitivity of these signs was variable (specificity 61-99 and 43-100 respectively and sensitivity 14-90 and 12-85). Tachypnoea had a better sensitivity in younger children (below 11 months) especially when the cut off value was 50, not 60 breaths per minute. Interesting data about tachypnoea came from one of the analyzed observational studies of 423 children living at an altitude of 3750 m in the Peruvian Andes who had acute respiratory infections (Reuland 1991). Compared with other studies of children living at lower altitudes, the presence of tachypnoea was relatively nonspecific as a predictor of radiographically determined pneumonia or of hypoxemia, especially in infants. Authors suggested that case management algorithms developed in low-altitude regions may have to be modified for high-altitude settings. Specificity of tachypnoea was variable between studies. This observations and use of different cut off points for diagnosis makes tachypnoea an unreliable indicator for oxygen therapy in children with pneumonia. Sensitivity and specificity of chest indrawings were very variable. Tachypnoea, grunting in young infants and severe chest in-drawing are parameters suggested by the WHO as an indicators for oxygen therapy (WHO 1993).

Data from these reviews showed that the three signs mentioned above, considered individually, have all been shown to be very non-specific in determining the presence of hypoxemia. The presence of crepitations on auscultation during admission to hospital was shown to have a good sensitivity (50-93) but lower specificity in most of studies (12-92). With exclusion of one study the presence of nasal flaring showed consistently good both sensitivity (48-98) and specificity (54-98). A summary presenting range of minimum to maximum sensitivity and specificity for each of the parameters discussed above as markers of hypoxia is shown in table 2.

Table 2. Sensitivity and specificity of clinical signs as indicators of hypoxemia in lower respiratory tract infections in children (data presented as minimum to maximum value from 12 observational studies)

Clinical sign	Sensitivity (%)	Specificity (%)
Cyanosis	5-74	75-100
Difficulty in feeding	28-71	60-99
Grunting	14-90	61-99
Altered mental status	12-85	43-100
Tachypnoea	16-90	24-100
Chest indrawing	35-98	7-94
Crepitations	50-93	12-92
Nasal flaring	48-98	54-98*

*Data from 11 studies (data from Usen 1999 not included)

In view of variability of data authors of this review concluded that:

> "there is still no clinical sign, model or score system that accurately identifies hypoxemic children. The measurement of SaO2 is still a particularly important test for physicians to make the correct decision regarding whether or not to give oxygen supplementation to infants and children with lower respiratory tract infections".

2.7. Comparison of Different Methods of Oxygen Delivery

In the hospital setting oxygen can be delivered to the patient by nasal cannulas, head box or face mask. First reports about advantages and disadvantages of different modes of delivery to pneumonia sufferers were published by Prendergast in 1927. Up to now there are 3 randomized controlled studies in children comparing effects of oxygen delivery via nasal prongs and nasopharyngeal catheter (Muhe 1997, Muhe 1998, Weber 1995) and only 1 quasi-RCT study comparing 4 different delivery modes (Kumar 1997). The latter study describes the efficacy and tolerance of oxygen delivery via: head box, face mask, nasopharyngeal catheter and twin-holed pre-nasal catheter in 80 children below five years of age presenting with acute respiratory distress who required oxygen to achieve a PaO2 of 60 mmHg. Children were assigned to receive oxygen administered by all four methods for 15 minutes in a pre-determined sequence. Efficacy of oxygen therapy was assessed by analysis of arterial blood gas and arterial oxygen saturation (SaO_2). Acceptability in terms of child comfort was assessed by a tolerance score as perceived by the mother. It was found that the face mask group presented lower treatment failures (failure to achieve a PaO2 > 60 mmHg) than the nasopharyngeal catheter group (OR 0.20; 95% CI 0.05 to 0.88). This result was highly significant. Frequency of treatment failure in the head box group was also fewer than in the nasopharyngeal catheter group (OR 0.40; 95%CI 0.13 to 1.12). The head box and nasal cannula were the best tolerated methods for delivery oxygen. The three randomized studies by Muhe (1997 and 1998) and Weber (1995) did not show significant differences in the effectiveness of nasal prongs in comparison with nasopharyngeal catheter, measured as the risk of treatment failure (OR 0.96; 95% CI 0.48 to 1.93). Side effects assessment showed nasal obstruction significantly less frequent in the nasal prongs group than in the nasopharyngeal catheter group. (OR 0.17; 95% CI 0.07 to 0.39). Significant side effects were not noted. Above data showed that there is currently not enough evidence to suggest superiority of one method of oxygen delivery over another.

Current Clinical Guidelines

Based on existing evidence there are currently three guidelines, published by the British Thoracic Society, available regarding use of oxygen in pneumonia:

1) Guideline for the Management of Community Acquired Pneumonia (CAP) in Childhood (British Thoracic Society 2002)

In this document hypoxemia is mentioned as a key indication for a child with pneumonia to be hospitalized. The Guideline Development Group mentioned results of a prospective study from Zambia where the risk of death from pneumonia was significantly increased when hypoxemia was present (Smyth 1998). Hypoxia was present in 55 from 158 (35%) children younger than 5 years admitted to district hospital. It was found that the likelihood of death was significantly increased in those children with low oxygen saturation ($p = 0.021$) and poor nutrition ($p = 0.007$). The Guideline recommends that infants and children with saturation < 92% or cyanosis should be hospitalized and treated with oxygen given by nasal cannulas, head box, or face mask to maintain oxygen saturation above 92%. During oxygen therapy the child should have at least 4 hourly observations including oxygen saturation.

2) Guidelines for the Management of Community Acquired Pneumonia in Adults (British Thoracic Society 2009)

The guideline states that every adult patient with pneumonia admitted to hospital should receive appropriate oxygen therapy. Decision about hospitalization should be based mainly on severity assessment using CURB65 criteria (confusion, raised urea, tachypnoea, low blood pressure and age > 65 years). Although measured hypoxia is not used directly in these criteria, confusion and tachypnoea may be indirect indicators. The guideline mentions low oxygen saturation (< 94%) in patients with CAP as an adverse prognostic feature and also an indication for oxygen therapy which will usually require urgent referral to hospital. Therefore the guideline suggests that pulse oximetry, with appropriate training, should be available to general practitioners and others responsible for the assessment of patients in the out-of-hours setting, for the assessment of severity and oxygen requirement in patients with CAP and other acute respiratory illnesses. After admission to hospital oxygen therapy should be provided with monitoring of oxygen saturations and inspired oxygen concentration with the aim to maintain ($PaO2$) $\geq$ 8 kPa and oxygen saturation ($SpO2$) 94–98%. High concentrations of oxygen can safely be given to patients who are not at risk of hypercapnic respiratory failure.

3) Emergency Oxygen Use in Adult Patients (British Thoracic Society 2008)

Pneumonia is listed there amongst other serious illnesses requiring moderate levels of supplemental oxygen but only if the patient is hypoxemic. It is suggested that initial oxygen therapy should be provided by nasal cannulas at 2–6 l/min or simple face mask at 5–10 l/min aiming to achieve a saturation within a target range of 94–98%. Patients who have co-existing chronic obstructive pulmonary disease (COPD) or other risk factors for hypercapnic respiratory failure should be commenced with a reservoir mask at 10–15 l/min aiming to achieve lower saturation than in otherwise healthy subjects (88-92%) to avoid possible decrease in respiratory "hypoxic drive" in that group of patients.

Summary

Oxygen is effective in treating hypoxemia in patients with pneumonia. The most reliable way of assessing for presence of hypoxia is measurement of partial oxygen pressure in blood or arterial oxygen saturation. There is no clinical sign, model or score system which accurately identifies hypoxemic patients. Cyanosis is the clinical sign with the highest specificity in detection of hypoxia. The other analyzed clinical signs have more variable specificity and sensitivity but still can be used with caution as indicators of hypoxia if direct measurements (PaO2 and SaO2) cannot be performed. It is at present unclear which of the non-invasive oxygen delivery methods is most suitable for treatment of hypoxemia. All methods are safe with no significant side effects reported in quoted observational studies. Decision about choosing the best method of oxygen therapy for individual patients is based on availability, patient tolerability and cost.

3. Chest Physiotherapy

The value of chest physical therapy as supportive treatment of patients hospitalised with acute pneumonia has been controversial. The British Thoracic Society guidelines for managing pneumonia in childhood stated that chest physical therapy is not beneficial and should not be performed in children with pneumonia (British Thoracic Society Standards of Care Committee 2002).

Effects of chest physiotherapy on outcome of pneumonia in adults have been systematically reviewed (Yang M 2010). Six RCTs (434 participants) appraised four types of chest physiotherapy (conventional chest physiotherapy; osteopathic manipulative treatment (which includes paraspinal inhibition, rib raising and myofascial release); active cycle of breathing techniques (which include active breathing control, thoracic expansion exercises and forced expiration techniques); and positive expiratory pressure). None of the physiotherapies (versus no physiotherapy or placebo) improved mortality rates of adults with pneumonia. Conventional chest physiotherapy (versus no physiotherapy), active cycle of breathing techniques (versus no physiotherapy) and osteopathic manipulative treatment (versus placebo) did not increase the cure rate or chest X-ray improvement rate. Osteopathic manipulative treatment (versus placebo) and positive expiratory pressure (versus no physiotherapy) reduced mean duration of hospital stay by 2.0 days (mean difference (MD) -2.0 days, 95% CI -3.5 to -0.6) and 1.4 days (MD -1.4 days, 95% CI -2.8 to -0.0), respectively.

Conventional chest physiotherapy and active cycle of breathing techniques did not. Positive expiratory pressure (versus no physiotherapy) reduced fever duration (MD -0.7 day, 95% CI -1.4 to -0.0). Osteopathic manipulative treatment did not. Osteopathic manipulative treatment (versus placebo) was associated with a reduced duration of intravenous (MD -2.1 days, 95% CI -3.4 to -0.9) and total antibiotic treatment (MD -1.9 days, 95% CI -3.1 to -0.7).

4. Supportive Therapy with Medication

4.1 Steroid Therapy

Steroids influence immune regulation and have effects on carbohydrate metabolism, protein catabolism, electrolyte balance and stress response. They are used therapeutically for treating inflammatory diseases of the bowel (colitis), joints (arthritis), skin (dermatitis) and lungs (pneumonia or asthma). Functionally, steroids act partly by inducing anti-inflammatory mediators, which repress inflammatory genes (Adcock 2000). Two previous randomised controlled trials showed that intravenous steroids given for at least 3 days may influence symptoms of severe pneumonia (See table 3). One trial showed that duration of ventilation in dexamethasone treated patients with bronchiolitis was significantly reduced. This finding is in contradiction to other trials using oral steroids in bronchiolitis: A systematic review summarized three double blind randomised placebo-controlled trials including a total of 705 patients (two using oral dexamethasone for 1 to 3 days and one using oral prednisolone for 3 days) which found no difference between groups in outcomes like respiratory rate, oxygen saturation, severity scores or duration of hospital stay (Panickar 2008).

Steroids have however been found to be a very important part of treatment of Pneumocystis jiroveci (PJP) pneumonia in patients with HIV infection. Six studies were included in a systematic review and meta-analysis of this topic (Briel 2006). Trials were considered eligible for this review if they compared corticosteroids to placebo or usual care in HIV-infected patients with PJP in addition to baseline treatment with trimethoprim-sulfamethoxazole, pentamidine or dapsone-trimethoprim, used random allocation, and reported mortality data. Risk ratios for overall mortality for adjunctive corticosteroids were 0.56 (95% confidence interval [CI], 0.32-0.98) at 1 month and 0.68 (95% CI, 0.50-0.94) at 3-4 months of follow-up. To prevent 1 death, numbers needed to treat are 9 patients in a setting without highly active antiretroviral therapy (HAART) available, and 23 patients with HAART available. Only the 3 largest trials provided data on the need for mechanical ventilation with a risk ratio of 0.38 (95% CI, 0.20-0.73) in favour of adjunctive corticosteroids.

Table 3. Results of randomised controlled trials of steroids in patients with lower respiratory tract infection (not due to Pneumoscystis jiroveci)

Trial design	Participants	Result	Conclusion	References
An open label, prospective, randomized controlled study	31 hospitalized patients with community acquired pneumonia, 15 patients given prednisolone 40mg once a day intravenously for 3 days and 16 patients managed without steroids.	Both groups demonstrated similar baseline characteristics and length of hospital stay, and yet a shorter duration of IV antibiotics was observed in the steroid group ($p < 0.05$). In addition, vital signs were stabilized earlier in the steroid group ($p < 0.05$).	In moderate–severe CAP, administration of corticosteroids promotes resolution of clinical symptoms and reduces the duration of intravenous antibiotic therapy.	Mikami 2007
Double blind randomised placebo controlled trial	48 patients hospitalised with severe pneumonia, 24 patients were allocated to intravenous hydrocortisone 200mg bolus followed by 10mg/h for 7 days, 24 to placebo.	By study day 8, steroid treated patients had, compared with control subjects, a significant improvement in PaO_2:FIO_2-ratio ($p = 0.002$) and chest radiograph score ($p = 0.0001$), and a significant reduction in C-reactive protein levels ($p=0.01$), MODS-score ($p=0.003$), and delayed septic shock ($p=0.001$). Hydrocortisone treatment was associated with a significant reduction in length of hospital stay ($p = 0.03$) and mortality ($p = 0.009$).	Prolonged low-dose hydrocortisone infusion may hasten resolution of pneumonia and prevent the development of sepsis-related complications.	Confalonieri 2005
Randomised placebo controlled trial	Included were patients with respiratory syncytial virus lower respiratory tract infection. Thirty seven patients received dexamethasone (0.15 mg/kg 6 hourly for 48 hours) and 45 received placebo.	There was no difference in duration of mechanical ventilation, length of stay in the pediatric intensive care unit and in hospital, and the duration of supplemental oxygen administration. In patients with bronchiolitis the duration of mechanical ventilation was 4.3 days shorter in the dexamethasone group than in the placebo group (4.9 v 9.2 days, 95% CI −7.8 to −0.8, $p=0.02$) and the duration of supplemental oxygen was 3.6 days shorter (7.7 v 11.3 days, 95% CI −8.0 to −0.1, $p=0.048$).	Dexamethasone had no beneficial effect in patients mechanically ventilated for RSV-LRTI but was found to have a beneficial effect in patients with bronchiolitis.	Van Woensel 2003
Randomised placebo controlled trial	Patients with severe pneumonia were included. Out of thirty patients recruited, 14 patients received 10mg/kg hydrocortisone which was given intravenously once 30 min before antibiotic administration.	Mortality and length of stay on the intensive care uni was not different between groups.	A single dose of hydrocortisone has not been shown to influence outcome in pneumona	Marik 1993

4.2. Granulocyte Colony Stimulating Factor Treatment

Endogenous granulocyte colony-stimulating factor (G-CSF), produced by endothelial cells, fibroblasts, monocytes and macrophages, plays a central role in polymorphonuclear (PMN) cell bone marrow release, proliferation, differentiation and intracellular microbial killing. In addition G-CSF has a marked inhibitory effect on PMN cell apoptosis in vitro resulting in prolonged survival. In healthy volunteers a profound inhibition of neutrophil apoptosis and an increased neutrophil activation after a single dose of G-CSF has been observed. In addition G-CSF caused an enhanced release of the cytokine antagonists sTNF-p55 and IL-1R (Droemann 2006). In various animal models of infection, multiple studies have shown that G-CSF can augment host response to a variety of infectious organisms with reduced mortality (Huber 2002). In experimental animal pneumonia G-CSF accelerates the clearance of pathogens from the lungs, by increasing the number and/or function of neutrophils. In an animal model of pulmonary sepsis, Karzai et al (Karzai 1999) demonstrated that the prophylactic application of G-CSF was beneficial in rats infected with *Staphylococcus aureus,* resulting in increased bacterial clearance and decreased death, whereas in *Escherichia coli* pneumonia, G-CSF paradoxically decreased circulating neutrophil counts and increased mortality. In this context Hollenstein et al. (Hollenstein 2000) demonstrated a downregulation of the G-CSF receptor (CD114) by endotoxin, possibly decreasing the G-CSF response.

A recent systematic review (Cheng AC 2007) identified six studies with a total of 2018 people reporting on the effects of use of G-CSF. G-CSF use appeared to be safe with no increase in the incidence of total serious adverse events (pooled odds ratio (OR) 0.91; 95% confidence interval (CI): 0.73 to 1.14) or organ dysfunction. However, the use of G-CSF was not associated with improved 28-day mortality (pooled OR 0.81; 95% CI: 0.52 to 1.27). There is therefore no current evidence supporting the routine use of G-CSF in the treatment of pneumonia.

4.3 Surfactant Application

In any episode of pneumonia, secondary surfactant deficiency may develop through two processes; surfactant inactivation (Rudiger 2001) and peroxidation (Bouhafs 1999; Bouhafs 2004). An autopsy study of neonates who died from Group B Streptococcus sepsis confirmed that most of them had surfactant deficiency or dysfunction (Payne 1988). Deficiency or deranged composition of surfactant has also been noted in infants beyond the first few days of life and even older children with severe bacterial pneumonia (Le Vine 1996). It may be that the surfactant pool in early neonatal life is not as large as later on (for example after two weeks of age) and this may potentially affect the severity of illness in these infants with pneumonia. Evidence on the possible role of surfactant in neonatal bacterial pneumonia is provided by animal studies. In animal models of Group B streptococci pneumonia, surfactant is reported to have immunomodulating effects (Talati 2001). The addition of surfactant with or without concurrent administration of immunoglobulin (Herting 1994; Herting 1999) seems to enhance bacterial clearance. In a study investigating the role of specific neutralizing antibodies to bacterial pneumonia, the antibodies were effective only when surfactant is added (Gan 2001). Along with other supportive treatment and antibiotics, surfactant therapy may be useful in the treatment of neonatal bacterial pneumonia. The postulated mechanisms of action are the reversal of surfactant inactivation that is a feature of bacterial pneumonia and local immunomodulating effects. A report of two ex-preterm infants with ARDS secondary to Chlamydia pneumonia provides the earliest human evidence on possible benefits of surfactant during bacterial pneumonia. The diagnoses were made from the clinical presentation, chest x-ray appearances, Chlamydia specific antigen from tracheal aspirates and isolation of the microorganism (in one infant). Both infants responded to surfactant administration and survived without chronic lung disease (Harms 1994). Other types of respiratory distress, for example, secondary to respiratory syncytial virus (RSV) infections have also been shown to respond to surfactant therapy (Ventre 2006). However, there is concern that certain types of surfactant appear to promote the growth of specific bacterial species (Rauprich 2000). Furthermore, there is the suggestion that surfactant administration may be associated with pulmonary haemorrhage (Raju 1993; Soll 1999). In addition, there are the risks associated with initial surfactant instillation including brief period of hypoxia, hypotension as well as altered cerebral haemodynamics (Cowan 1991; Kaiser 2004).

Ventilator-associated pneumonia (VAP) has, despite use of antibiotics, a 30-60% mortality. In addition to preventative strategies supportive measures are required to improve outcome. The first double-blind randomised controlled trial using surfactant in VAP selected patients from those requiring mechanical ventilation with presence of new or worsening infiltrate, purulent sputum or tracheal secretions, and either fever or leukocytosis/leukopenia. Excluded were patients with pneumocystic jiroveci pneumonia, multiorgan failure or ARDS. Twenty-two patients were randomised, with 8 receiving Exosurf. There was no detected difference in outcome between the saline-and Exosurf-treated patients in terms of days on ventilator, 30-day or hospital mortality (Baughman 2002).

5. Fluid Management

Supportive therapy with parenteral fluid has been recommended by the World Health Organization (WHO) for the management of severe and very severe pneumonia in children, especially in patients with hypoxaemia (WHO 1990). Guidelines for treating pneumonia in adults also contain advice on fluid management (BTS 2002). The objectives of fluid therapy include the replacement of fluid losses and both prevention and correction of electrolyte disturbances (Roberts 2001). The amount of fluid required is debatable as both dehydration and overhydration may adversely affect critically ill patients (Guppy 2005). Dehydration may result in hypovolemic shock, but overhydration may result in low sodium concentrations and pulmonary edema, which can aggravate hypoxaemia and increase mortality. There have been reports of an increase in antidiuretic hormone secretion in adults and children with lower respiratory tract infections. In some cases, the secretion of the hormone increased proportionally with the involvement of pulmonary tissue (Dreyfuss 1988). While the pathophysiological basis is not fully understood, the main mechanisms proposed are dilution of extracellular fluid because of impaired free-water excretion and increased urinary sodium losses. However, some studies suggest that hyponatremia arises either as a result of an appropriate physiological response of antidiuretic hormone to restore extracellular fluid volume at the expense of hypo-osmolarity, or as a result of hormonal activity that is inappropriate to both osmolarity and fluid volume status (Duke 2002; von Vigier 2001).

Although hyponatremia has been clearly documented in conditions such as meningitis (von Vigier 2001), encephalitis (Mc Junkin 2001) and septicemia (Jensen 1999), water retention is also believed to be present in acute pneumonia (Dhawan 1992; Shann 1985). Patient data on actual changes in body water compartments and plasma volume have shown that extracellular water and plasma volume were moderately increased in severe and very severe pneumonia in children. Such increases were correlated with better oxygenation (Singhi 2005). These findings suggest that the fluid restriction in hypoxaemic patients with severe pneumonia should occur after the correction of hypoxaemia. (Dhawan 1992; Gozal 1990; Singhi 2005).

Literature search could identify only one randomized controlled trial of different fluid regimens in acute lung injury (National Heart, Lung, and Blood Institute Acute Respiratory Distress Syndrome (ARDS) Clinical Trials Network 2006). It compared a conservative and a liberal strategy of fluid management using explicit protocols applied for seven days in 1000 patients with acute lung injury. During the study, the seven-day cumulative fluid balance was –136+/-491 ml in the conservative-strategy group, as compared with 6992 +/-502 ml in the liberal-strategy group (P<0.001). For patients who were in shock at baseline, the cumulative seven-day fluid balance was 2904+/-1008 ml in the conservative-strategy group and 10,138 +/-922 ml in the liberal-strategy group (P<0.001). For patients who were not in shock at baseline, the cumulative fluid balance was −1576 +/-519 ml in the conservative-strategy group and 5287 +/-576 ml in the liberal-strategy group (P<0.001).The primary end point was death at 60 days. Secondary end points included the number of ventilator-free days and organ-failure-free days and measures of lung physiology. The rate of death at 60 days was 25.5 percent in the conservative-strategy group and 28.4 percent in the liberal-strategy group (P=0.30; 95 percent confidence interval for the difference, -2.6 to 8.4 percent). The mean (+/-SE) cumulative fluid balance during the first seven days was -136+/-491 ml in the conservative-strategy group and 6992+/-502 ml in the liberal-strategy group (P<0.001). As compared with the liberal strategy, the conservative strategy improved the oxygenation index ([mean airway pressure x the ratio of the fraction of inspired oxygen to the partial pressure of arterial oxygen]x100) and the lung injury score and increased the number of ventilator-free days (14.6+/-0.5 vs. 12.1+/-0.5, P<0.001) and days not spent in the intensive care unit (13.4+/-0.4 vs. 11.2+/-0.4, P<0.001) during the first 28 days but did not increase the incidence or prevalence of shock during the study or the use of dialysis during the first 60 days (10 percent vs. 14 percent, P=0.06). The conclusion of the authors was: Although there was no significant difference in the primary outcome of 60-day mortality, the conservative strategy of fluid management improved lung function and shortened the duration of mechanical ventilation and intensive care without increasing nonpulmonary-organ failures. These results supported the use of a conservative strategy of fluid management in patients with acute lung injury.

6. Micronutrient Supplementation in Pneumonia

In a double-blind, placebo-controlled randomized trial, HIV-infected children (4–24 mo) who were hospitalized with diarrhea or pneumonia were enrolled (n = 118) and given a daily dose of a multi-micronutrient supplement (containing vitamins A, B complex, C, D, E, and folic acid, as well as copper, iron, and zinc at levels based on recommended daily allowances) or a placebo until discharge from the hospital. Among children admitted with pneumonia those who received the supplement had a 20% shorter duration of hospitalization (Mda 2010). The results of this trial underscore the importance of assessment of each component of this mixture of supplements for its effect on outcome of pneumonia.

6.1. Vitamin A

The effect of Vitamin A application in children with pneumonia has been reviewed previously (Wu 2005). The systematic review revealed six trials involving 1740 children. There was no significant reduction in mortality associated with pneumonia in children treated with vitamin A compared to those who were not (pooled odds ratio (OR) 1.29; 95% confidence interval (CI) 0.62 to 2.69). Also, there was no statistically significant difference in duration of hospital stay (mean difference (MD) 0.08; 95% CI -0.43 to 0.59). Vitamin A was associated with a 39% reduction in antibiotic first line failure (OR 0.65; 95% CI 0.42 to 1.01). Disease severity after supplementary high-dose vitamin A was significantly worse compared with placebo. However, low-dose vitamin A significantly reduced the recurrence rate of bronchopneumonia (OR 0.12; 95% CI 0.03 to 0.46). Moderately dosed vitamin A significantly reduced the time to remission of signs in children with normal serum retinol (> 200 ug/L). The evidence does not suggest a significant reduction in mortality, measures of morbidity, nor an effect on the clinical course of pneumonia with vitamin A adjunctive treatment in children with non-measles pneumonia.

6.2. Vitamin C

There is a paucity of studies using vitamin C as supportive treatment in pneumonia. A recent Cochrane review (Hemilä 2007) identified after an extensive search two therapeutic trials involving 197 pneumonia patients (Mochalkin 1970, Hunt 1994). These two trials examined the effect of vitamin C on patients with pneumonia (Mochalkin 1970) or pneumonia and bronchitis (Hunt 1994). Hunt et al. found a 85% lower mortality in the vitamin C group compared with the placebo group, but this comparison was based on six cases only. There was statistically marginal significance of overall benefit on the respiratory score with vitamin C, but in a subgroup analysis based on the baseline severity of disease, the benefit was restricted to patients who were most severely ill when admitted to the hospital. These most severely ill patients had substantially lower vitamin C plasma levels compared with the less ill patients. In the less ill patients, there was no difference between the trial arms. Mochalkin's study had three trial arms: control, low vitamin C and high vitamin C. Because of their protocol, the mean vitamin C dose of the higher dose arm was exactly double that of the lower dose arm, although the dosage ranges within both vitamin C arms varied and overlapped. There was a statistically highly significant decrease in length of hospital stay in the higher vitamin C dose arm compared with the lower dose arm. Mochalkin reported the proportion of participants with no fever after seven days and with normalisation of the CXR in 10 days. For both outcomes, the vitamin C arms fared significantly better than the control arm. The number needed to treat (NNT) was around five for these two outcomes compared to the control group. In Mochalkin's study the duration of recovery was reduced from 23.7 days in the control group by 4.6 days (19%) in the low-dose vitamin C arm and by 8.6 days (36%) in the high-dose vitamin C arm. Since the mean vitamin C dose in the high vitamin C arm was exactly twice the mean of the lower vitamin C arm, the linearity in this response was unusual. Both therapeutic trials used CXR when evaluating patients, but neither provided a well-defined case definition of pneumonia; nor of lower respiratory tract infection. However, therapeutic vitamin C supplementation may be reasonable for pneumonia patients who have low vitamin C plasma levels because its cost and risks are low.

6. 3. Vitamin D

Vitamin D has multiple effects on the immune system and is an inducer of antimicrobial peptides as summarized in a previous review, which is in its essential parts summarized below (Eisenhut 2009). Most data from systematic research refer to its effect on mycobacterium tuberculosis infection including pulmonary tuberculosis. Historical data suggested the successful use of calciferol inducing or supplementing treatment in patients with tuberculosis from the pre-chemotherapy era (Macrae 1946, Dowling 1946). Anecdotal evidence suggested successful treatment of tuberculosis patients with vitamin D containing cod liver oil in the middle of the 19th century (Davies 1985). Sunlight exposure which induces vitamin D production in skin cells was found to be successful in treatment of lupus vulgaris (tuberculosis of the skin) with a 95% success rate, a principle for which the Nobel prize was awarded to Finsen in 1903 (Zasloff 2006). Early research showed that in conjunction with an unknown factor present in serum calcitriol caused a threefold slowing of intra-macrophageal bacillary replication from a generation time of a mean of 23.5 hours to a mean of 71.8 hours in human macrophages (Crowle 1987). This was achieved at a concentration of calcitriol of 4 microgram/ml as opposed to 2.6 to 7.0×10^{-5} microgram/ml in the normal circulating range. The antimycobacterial mechanism was found to involve the induction of expression of multiple antimicrobial peptides mediated by the vitamin D receptor complex in keratinocytes, monocytes and neutrophils (Wang 2004). An important antimicrobial peptide induced by calcitriol in phagocytes found to kill mycobacterium tuberculosis within phagocytic vacuoles is LL-37, which is also chemoattractant for monocytes and macrophages (Liu 2006). Recent work indicated that interaction of pathogen-associated molecular patterns shed from the cell wall of mycobacterium tuberculosis interact with the toll like receptor 2/1 dimer pair on the macrophage triggering upregulation of expression of both the CYP 2761 and VDR. This permits the macrophage to internalise serum vitamin D binding protein-bound 25 hydroxy vitamin D from the extracellular fluid by facilitated endocytosis where it becomes substrate for the upregulated CYP2761. Calcitriol then transactivates the endogenous defensive gene, cathelicidin and thus leads to expression of LL-37 leading to killing of intracellular mycobacterium tuberculosis. Extracellular 25 hydroxy vitamin D was hereby as or more effective than equimolar concentrations of calcitriol in inducing LL-37 production despite its much lower affinity to VDR (Adams 2007). Calcitriol induced antimicrobial activity was completely inhibited in the presence of small interfering RNA against mRNA of LL-37 (cathelicidin) (Liu 2007). This proved that in the human monocytic cell line THP-1 antimicrobial peptide LL-37 induction was the only mechanism of antimycobacterial activity. Application of a single dose of oral vitamin D in a double blind randomised controlled trial in 192 adults resulted in an increased ability of participants whole blood to restrict BCG-lux luminescence in vitro (Martineau 2007). The 24-hour luminescence ratio was 20.4% lower for individuals allocated to vitamin D compared with those allocated to placebo (0.57 vs 0.71 respectively; 95% CI for difference, 0.01-0.25; p=0.03). The size of the effect observed probably explains why in a small trial (n=8) of UV-B induced increase (approximately doubling) of serum Vitamin D levels no effect on BCG-lux luminescence was observed (Yesudian 2008). A systematic review identified 14 prospective clinical studies in which vitamin D had been administered in patients with pulmonary tuberculosis (Martineau 2007). Three studies were randomised controlled trials (RCT's) and the others case series. None of the RCT's which had between 23 and 60 participants demonstrated a therapeutic response. A study conducted in Indonesia in patients with moderately advanced pulmonary tuberculosis demonstrated that patients given vitamin D had a higher rate of sputum conversion and an increased radiological improvement compared with the placebo group (Nursyam 2006). In a randomized, double-blind, placebo controlled trial in TB clinics at a demographic surveillance site in Guinea-Bissau investigators included 365 adult patients with TB starting antituberculosis treatment; 281 completed the 12-month follow up. The intervention was 100,000 IU of cholecalciferol or placebo at inclusion and again 5 and 8 months after the start of treatment. The primary outcome was reduction in a clinical severity score (TB score) for all patients with pulmonary TB. The secondary outcome was 12-month mortality. No serious adverse effects were reported; mild hypercalcemia was rare and present in both arms. Reduction in TB score and sputum smear conversion rates did not differ among patients treated with vitamin D or placebo. Overall mortality was 15% (54 of 365) at 1 year of follow-up and similar in both arms (30 of 187 for vitamin D treated and 24 of 178 for placebo; relative risk, 1.19 [0.58–1.95]) (Wejse 2009).

6.4. Zinc

Zinc is involved in all major biochemical pathways and multiple cellular processes. Zinc is an essential contributing factor to immunocompetence and mucosal integrity (Aggett 1995; Bhatangar 2004). Zinc deficiency is associated with decreased immunocompetence (Golden 1995; Sazawal 1997; Shankar 1998) and increased incidence of serious infectious diseases, such as malaria, skin infections, diarrhea and respiratory tract infections (Black 2001; Lopez 1989; Murray 1996). Four high quality randomised controlled trials have so far been conducted to investigate the effect of zinc supplementation on the course of pneumonia.

In a double-blind, placebo-controlled clinical trial, children aged 2–35 mo with severe (n = 149) or nonsevere (n = 2479) pneumonia defined according to criteria established by the World Health Organization were randomly assigned to receive zinc (10 mg for children aged 2–11 mo, 20 mg for children aged 12 mo) or placebo daily for 14 d as an adjuvant to antibiotics. One of 5 children did not respond adequately to antibiotic treatment; the odds ratios between zinc and placebo groups for treatment failure were 0.95 (95% CI: 0.78, 1.2) for nonsevere pneumonia and 0.97 (95% CI: 0.42, 2.2) for severe pneumonia. There was no difference in time to recovery between zinc and placebo groups for nonsevere (median: 2 d; hazard ratio: 1.0; 95% CI: 0.96, 1.1) or severe (median: 4 d; hazard ratio: 1.1; 95% CI: 0.79, 1.5) pneumonia. Regurgitation or vomiting 15 min after supplementation was observed more frequently among children in the zinc group than among those in the placebo group during the supplementation period (37% compared with 13%; odds ratio: 0.25; 95% CI: 0.20, 0.30). (Valentiner-Branth 2010).

In another randomized, double-blind, placebo-controlled clinical trial conducted at the Christian Medical College Hospital, a teaching hospital in Tamilnadu, India children aged 2–23 mo (n=299) were randomly assigned to receive a 10-mg tablet of zinc sulfate or placebo twice a day during hospitalization. Etiology modified the treatment effect of zinc on the length of the hospital stay [hazard ratio (HR) for interaction term: 0.52; 95% CI: 0.31, 0.91; P = 0.022]. In the 72 suspected bacterial cases, the median length of hospitalization was 20 h longer in the zinc-supplemented group than in the placebo group (87.3 and 68.3 h, respectively; HR: 0.56; 95% CI:0.34, 0.93; P=0.025). The treatment effect was not modified in the suspected nonbacterial cases of pneumonia.(Coles 2007).

In a double-blind placebo-controlled clinical trial in Matlab Hospital, Bangladesh, 270 children aged 2–23 months were randomised to receive elemental zinc (20 mg per day) or placebo, plus the hospital's standard antimicrobial management, until discharge. The group receiving zinc had reduced duration of severe pneumonia (relative hazard [RH]=0·70, 95% CI 0·51–0·98), including duration of chest indrawing (0·80, 0·61–1·05), respiratory rate more than 50 per min (0·74, 0·57–0·98), and hypoxia (0·79, 0·61–1·04), and overall hospital duration (0·75, 0·57–0·99). The mean reduction is equivalent to one hospital day for both severe pneumonia and time in hospital. All effects were greater when children with wheezing were omitted from the analysis (Brooks 2004).

In a double-blind, randomized controlled trial, children aged 9 mo–15 y who were admitted to the Infectious Diseases Hospital in Calcutta with clinically severe measles accompanied by pneumonia and who had been ill for ≤ 7 d were randomly assigned to receive zinc (20 mg, in elemental form as acetate, twice daily for 6 d) or a placebo. Time-to-event analysis using the Cox proportional hazards model (42 in the zinc group and 43 in the placebo group) showed that the time needed for the resolution of fever and tachypnea, the return of appetite, and the achievement of a "much improved" or "cured" status was not different between the 2 groups. A high proportion of children had low serum retinal and zinc concentrations. Improvement in serum zinc and retinol concentrations after 6 d of treatment was not different between the 2 groups. (Mahalanabis 2002).

7. Protein and Calorie Supplements

Serum albumin is used to measure the nutritional status, as the rate of albumin synthesis can be decreased by malnutrition. However, this test may be inaccurate in patients with pneumonia as serum albumin levels can also be affected by infections. Hypoalbuminemia has been shown to be a risk factor for pneumonia in the elderly (Riquelme 1996). The only randomised controlled trial using food supplementation in lower respiratory tract infection used food as an incentive to improve compliance with medication in treatment of pulmonary tuberculosis. 265 patients were randomised. There was no significant difference in treatment success between groups even though patients on food incentives gained significantly more weight (Martins 2009).

8. Recommendations for Future Research

Implications for further Research

With regards to oxygen therapy a standardized definition of hypoxemia is required. This will need collection of cohort data of saturation values in healthy individuals living on different altitudes above sea level. Physiological effects of oxygen therapy may be wider than only correction of hypoxemia. There is no data comparing effects of oxygen therapy in non hypoxemic and hypoxemic patients with respiratory tract infections. Studies to identify the most effective, safest and most cost effective non invasive oxygen therapy methods are needed. There is no clear data how long oxygen therapy should be provided (end point definition) and there is also a lack of determinants for continuation of treatment after discharge from hospital. On the basis of its key role in induction of antimicrobial peptides the effect of vitamin D in bacterial pneumonia other than caused by Mycobacterium tuberculosis needs to be explored. Surfactant use in bacterial pneumonia is largely unexplored and merits on the basis of dramatic effects on surfactant deficient lung disease in prematurely born infants further research.

As a basis for progress in finding effective supportive medication for patients with pneumonia the basic underlying pathophysiology of its morbidity and mortality needs to be understood and targeted.

Inflammatory mediators can apart from adverse effect on the cardiovascular system causing septic shock in bacterial pneumonia contribute to morbidity and mortality by reduction of pulmonary fluid clearance and hence induction of hypoxia by pulmonary fluid accumulation in sepsis related pulmonary edema and pneumonia. Sodium and chloride transport across alveolar epithelia generates hereby the osmotic gradient enabling water absorption from the alveolar space (Matthay 2002). Future studies need to explore the use of hormones and synthetic or plant or animal generated compounds in up-regulating function and expression of ion transport systems involved in establishing this osmotic gradient. Examples are aldosterone and thyroxine which upregulate expression of the sodium potassium ATPase, which drives transepithelial sodium transport at the basolateral membrane of alveolar epithelial cells. Corticosteroids may also act on expression and function of ion transport systems and reduce expression of a wide range of inflammatory mediators involved in downregulation of ion transport system expression and function. This makes these hormones an attractive potential adjuvant supporting pulmonary fluid clearance. Targeted reversal of inhibition of ion channels like the epithelial sodium channel or the cystic fibrosis conductance regulator chloride channel in local or systemic inflammatory responses by inflammatory mediators (Eisenhut 2006) would require stereospecific changes in phosphorylation of ion channels, which should be subject of future investigations.

Conclusion

Undisputable cornerstones of supportive treatment of patients with pneumonia remain optimisation of oxygenation, and maintenance of adequate hydration and nutrition. The optimal dose and composition of each of these supportive treatments however has so far been inadequately investigated. Supportive treatment with medication showed promising results for bacterial pneumonia with prolonged treatment with steroids in small trials, which need to be confirmed in larger studies. Trials using supplementation with vitamin A or zinc did not show consistent benefit. For surfactant, fluid regimes, chest physiotherapy, vitamin C and D and protein and calorie supplements there has been a lack of investigations allowing any conclusion about influence on outcome and further research is required.

References

Adams, J. S., Liu, P.T., Chuu, R., Modlin, R.I., Hewison, M., (2007) Vitamin D in defense of the human immune response. *Ann. N.Y. Acad. Sci.* 1117; 94-105.

Adcock, I.M., Ito, K.. (2000). Molecular mechanisms of corticosteroid actions. *Monaldi Archives for Chest Disease* 256:66.

Aggett, P.J., Comerford, J.G. (1995). Zinc and human health. *Nutrition Reviews* 53:16-22.

Ayieko, P., English, M. (2006). In children aged 2-59 months with pneumonia, which clinical signs best predict hypoxaemia? *J. Tropical Paediatics* 52, 5: 307-310

Baughman, R.P., Henderson, R.F., Whitsett, J., Gunther, K.L., Keeton, D.A., Waide, J.J., Zaccardelli, D.S., Pattishall, E.N., Rashkin, M.C.(2002). Surfactant replacement for ventilator-associated pneumonia: A preliminary report. *Respiration* 69: 57-62.

Bhatangar, S., Natchu, U.C.(2004).Zinc in child health and disease. *Indian Journal of Pediatrics* 71(11):991-995.

Binger, M.W., Judd, E.S., Moore, A.B. (1928). Oxygen in the treatment of postoperative bronchopneumonia. *Arch Surg.* 17:1047-1050

Black, R.E., Sazawal, S.(2001). Zinc and childhood infectious diseases morbidity and mortality. *British Journal of Nutrition* 85(Suppl 2):125-129.

Bouhafs, R.K., Jarstrand, C.(1999).Lipid peroxidation of lung surfactant by bacteria. *Lung* 177:101-110.

Bouhafs, R.K., Jarstrand, C., Robertson, B. (2004).Lipid peroxidation of lung surfactant in experimental neonatal group B streptococcal pneumonia. *Lung* 182:61-72.

Briel M, Bucher HC, Boscacci R, Furrer H. (2006). Adjunctive corticosteroids for Pneumocystis jiroveci pneumonia in patients with HIV-infection.*Cochrane Database Syst. Rev.* ;3:CD006150.

British Thoracic Society Standards of Care Committee. (2002). BTS guidelines for the management of community acquired pneumonia in childhood. *Thorax* 57(Suppl1): 1-24.

British Thoracic Society Standards of Care Committee. BTS (2008). Emergency Oxygen Use in Adult Patients. *Thorax* 63, supplement VI

British Thoracic Society Standards of Care Committee. BTS (2009). Guidelines for the Management of Community Acquired Pneumonia in Adults. *Thorax* 64, Supplement III

Brooks, W.A., Yunus, M., Santosham, M., Wahed, M.A., Nahar, K., Yeasmin, S., Black, R.E. (2004). Zinc for severe pneumonia in very young children: double-blind placebo-controlled trial. *Lancet* 363: 1683–1688

Cheng, A.C., Stephens, D.P., Currie, B.J.(2007).Granulocyte-Colony Stimulating Factor (G-CSF) as an adjunct to antibiotics in the treatment of pneumonia in adults. *Cochrane Database of Systematic Reviews*, Issue 2. Art. No.: CD004400. DOI: 10.1002/14651858.CD004400.pub3.

Coles, C.L., Bose, A., Moses, P.D., Mathew, L., Agarwal, I., Mammen, T., Santosham, M. (2007). Infectious etiology modifies the treatment effect of zinc in severe pneumonia. *Am J Clin Nutr* 86:397– 403

Confalonieri, M., Urbino, R., Potena, A., Piatella, M., Parigi, P., Puccio, G., Porta, R.D., Giorgio, C., Blasi, F., Umberger, R., Meduri, G.U. (2005). Hydrocortisone infusion for severe community-acquired pneumonia. *Am.J.Resp.Crit. Care Med.* 171: 242-248.

Cowan, F., Whitelaw, A., Wertheim, D., Silverman, M. (1991). Cerebral blood flow velocity changes after rapid administration of surfactant. *Archives of Disease in Childhood* 66:1105-1109.

Crowle, A.J., Ross, E.J., May, M.H. (1987). Inhibiton by 1,25 $(OH)_2$ –Vitamin D_3 of the multiplication of virulent tubercle bacilli in cultured human macrophages. *Infection Immun.* 55: 2945-2950.

Davies, P.D.O. (1985). A possible link between vitamin D deficiency and impaired host defence to Mycobacterium tuberculosis. *Tubercle* 66: 301-306.

Dhawan, A., Narang, A., Singhi, S. (1992). Hyponatremia and the inappropriate ADH syndrome in pneumonia. *Annals of Tropical Paediatrics* 12:455-462.

Dreyfuss, D., Leviel, F., Rahmani, J., Coste, F. (1988).Acute infectious pneumonia is accompanied by latent vasopressin-dependent impairment of renal water excretion. *American Review of Respiratory Disease* 138:583-589.

Dowling, G.B., Prosser-Thomas, E.W. (1946) Treatment of lupus vulgaris with calciferol. *Lancet* 1: 919-922.

Droemann, D., Hansen, F., Aries, S.P., Braun, J., Zabel, P., Dalhoff, K., Schaaf, B. (2006). Neutrophil Apoptosis, Activation and anti-inflammatory cytokine response in granulocyte colony-stimulating factor-treated patients with community-acquired pneumonia. *Respiration* 73:340–346

Duke, T., Mokela, D., Frank, D., Michael, A., Paulo, T., Mgone, J., et al. (2002). Management of meningitis in children with oral fluid restriction or intravenous fluid at maintenance volumes: a randomised trial. *Annals of Tropical Paediatrics* 22:145-157.

Duke, T., Wandi, F., Jonathan, M., Matai, S., Kaupa, M., Saavu, M., Subhi, R., Peel D. (2008). Improved oxygen systems for childhood pneumonia: a multihospital effectiveness study in Papua New Guinea. *Lancet*. 372:1328-1333.

Dyke, T., Brown, N. (1994). Hypoxia in childhood pneumonia: better detection and more oxygen needed in developing countries. *BMJ*. 308:119-120,

Eisenhut, M.(2006). Changes in ion transport in inflammatory disease. *J Inflamm* 3:5

Eisenhut, M. (2009) The role of 1, 25 dihydroxy-vitamin D3 in immunity to infectious disease. *In Clinical Chemistry Research* [edited by] Brian H Mitchem and Charles L Sharnham. Nova Science Publishers, Inc. New York 221-239.

Gan, X., Jarstrand, C., Herting, E., Berggren, P., Robertson, B. (2001). Effect of surfactant and specific antibody on bacterial proliferation and lung function in experimental pneumococcal pneumonia. *International Journal of Infectious Diseases* 5:9-18.

Golden, M.H.N., Golden, B.E. (1995). Zinc and delayed hypersensitivity responses. *Nutrition Research Suppl* 1:700-709.

Gozal, D., Colin, A.A., Jaffe, M., Hochberg, Z.(1990). Water, electrolyte, and endocrine homeostasis in infants with bronchiolitis. *Pediatric Research* 27:204-209.

Guppy, M.P.B., Mickan, S.M., Del Mar, C.B. (2005). Advising patients to increase fluid intake for treating acute respiratory infections. *Cochrane Database of Systematic Reviews*, Issue 4. DOI: 10.1002/14651858.CD004419.pub2

Haldane, J.S. (1917). The therapeutic administration of oxygen. *B.M.J.* 10:181-183

Harms, K., Herting, E. (1994). Successful surfactant replacement therapy in two infants with ARDS due to chlamydial pneumonia. *Respiration* 61:348-352.

Hemilä, H., Louhiala, P. (2007). Vitamin C for preventing and treating pneumonia. *Cochrane Database of Systematic Reviews*, Issue 1.Art. No.: CD005532. DOI: 10.1002/14651858. CD005532.pub2.

Herting, E., Jarstrand, C., Rasool, O., Curstedt ,T., Sun, B., Robertson, B.(1994). Experimental neonatal group B streptococcal pneumonia: effect of a modified porcine surfactant on bacterial proliferation in ventilated near-term rabbits. *Pediatr. Res.* 36:784-791.

Herting, E., Gan, X., Rauprich, P., Jarstrand, C., Robertson, B. (1999). Combined treatment with surfactant and specific immunoglobulin reduces bacterial proliferation in experimental neonatal group B streptococcal pneumonia. *Am..J. Resp..Crit. Care Med.* 159(6):1862-1867.

Hollenstein, U., Homoncik, M., Stohlawetz, P.J., et al. (2000). Endotoxin down-modulates granulocyte colony-stimulating factor receptor (CD114) on human neutrophils. *J. Infect. Dis.* 182:343–346.

Huber, K., Dale, D.C., Liles, W.C. (2002). Therapeutic use of cytokines to modulate phagocyte function for the treatment of infectious diseases: current status of granulocyte colony-stimulating factor, granulocyte-macrophage colony-stimulatingfactor, macrophage colony-stimulating factor, and interferon-gamma. *J. Infect. Dis* 185: 1490–1501.

Hunt, C., Chakravorty, N.K., Annan, G., Habibzadeh, N., Schorah, C.J.(1994).The clinical effects of vitamin C supplementation in elderly hospitalised patients with acute respiratory infections. *Internat. J. Vit. Nutr. Res.* 64:212-219.

Jensen, A.G., Wachmann, C.H., Poulsen, K.B., Espersen, F., Scheibel, J., Skinhøj, P., et al. (1999). Risk factors for hospital-acquired Staphylococcus aureus bacteraemia. *Arch. Intern. Med.* 159:1437-1444.

Kaiser, J.R., Gauss, C.H., Williams, D.K. (2004). Surfactant administration acutely affects cerebral and systemic hemodynamics and gas exchange in very-low-birth-weight infants. *J. Pediatr.* 144:809-814.

Karzai, W., von Specht, B.U., Parent, C., et al.(1999). GCSF during *Escherichia coli* versus *Staphylococcus aureus* pneumonia in rats has fundamentally different and opposite effects. *Am. J. Resp. Crit. Care Med.* 159: 1377–1382.

Kumar, R.M., Kabra, S.K., Singh, M. (1997). Efficacy and acceptability of different modes of oxygen administration in children: implications for a community hospital. *Journal of Tropical Pediatrics* 43(1): 47–49

LeVine, A.M., Lotze, A., Stanley, S., Stroud, C., O'Donnell, R., Whitsett, J., et al. (1996). Surfactant content in children with inflammatory lung disease. *Crit. Care Med.* 24:1062-1067.

Liu, P.T., Stenger, S., Li, H., Wenzel, L., Tan, B.H., Krutzik, S.R., Ochoa, M.T., Schauber, J., Wu, K., Meinken, C., Kamen, D.L., Wagner, M., Bals, R., Stein-Meyer, A., Zuegel, U., Gallo, R.L., Eisenberg, D., Hewison, M., Hollis, B.W., Adams, J.S., Bloom, B.R., Modlin, R.L. (2006). Toll-like receptor triggering of a vitamin D-mediated human antimicrobial response. *Science* 311: 1770-1773.

Liu, P.T., Stenger, S., Tang, D.H., Modlin, R.L. (2007). Cutting edge: Vitamin D mediated human antimicrobial activity against Mycobacterium tuberculosis is independent on the induction of cathelicidin. *J. Immunol.*179: 2060-2063.

López de Romaña, G., Brown, K.H., Black, R.E., Kanashiro, H.(1989). Longitudinal studies of infectious diseases and physical growth of infants in Huascar, an underprivileged peri-urban community in Lima, Peru. *Am. J.Epidemiol.* 129:769-784.

Lozano, J.M. (2001). Epidemiology of hypoxaemia in children with acute lower respiratory infection. *Int. J. Tuberc. Lung Dis.* 5(6):496-504

Macrae, D.E. (1946). Calciferol treatment of lupus vulgaris. *Br. J. Dermatol.* 58: 333-338.

Mahalanabis, D., Chowdhury, A., Jana, S., Bhattacharya, M.K,, Chakrabarti, M.K,, Wahed, M.A., Khaled, M.A. (2002). Zinc supplementation as adjunct therapy in children with measles accompanied by pneumonia: a double-blind, randomized controlled trial. *Am. J. Clin. Nutr.* 76:604–607.

Marik, P., Kraus, P., Sribante, J., Havlik, I., Lipman, J., Johnson .(1993). Hydrocortisone and tumor necrosis factor in severe community-acquired pneumonia. A randomised controlled study. *Chest* 104: 389-392.

Martin, L. (1998). Oxygen therapy: the first 150 years. Available at: *http://www.lakesidepress.com/pulmonary/papers/ox-hist/ox-hist-intro.html Accessed 10 October 2010*

Martineau, A.R., Honecker, F.U., Wilkinson, R.J., Griffiths, C.J. (2007). Vitamin D in the treatment of pulmonary tuberculosis. *J. Steroid Biochem. Molec. Biol.* 103: 793-798.

Martineau, A.R., Wilkinson, R.J., Wilkinson, K.A., Newton, S.M., Kampmann, B., Hall, B.M., Packe, G.E., Davidson, R.N., Eldridge, S.M., Maunsell, Z.J., Rainbow, S.J., Bery, J.L., Griffiths, C.J. (2007). A single Dose of vitamin D enhances immunity to mycobacteria. *Am. J. Respir. Crit. Care Med.* 176: 208-213.

Martins, N., Morris, P., Kelly, P..M. (2009). Food incentives to improve completion of tuberculosis treatment: randomised controlled trial in Dili, Timor-Leste. *B.M.J.* 339: b4248.

Matthay, M.A., Folkesson, H.G., Clerici, C. (2002). Lung epithelial fluid transport and the resolution of pulmonary edema. *Physiol. Rev.* 82: 569-600

McJunkin, J.E., de los Reyes, E.C., Irazuzta, J.E., Caceres, M.J., Khan, R.R., Minnich, L.L., et al. (2001).La Crosse encephalitis in children. *N. E. J. M.* 344:801-807.

Mda, S., Van Raaij, I.M.A., De Villiers, F.P.R., MacIntyre, U.E., Kok F.J. (2010). Short-term micronutrient supplementation reduces the duration of pneumonia and diarrheal episodes in HIV-Infected children. *J.Nutr.* 140: 969–974.

Meltzer, S.J. (1917). The therapeutic value of oral rhytmic insufflation of oxygen. *J. A. M. A.* 6:1150-1156

Mikami, K., Suzuki, M., Kitagawa, H., Kawakami, M., Hirota, N., Yamaguchi, H., Narumoto, O., Kichikawa, Y., Kawai, M., Tashimo, H., Arai, H., Horiuchi, T., Sakamoto, Y. (2007). Efficacy of corticosteroids*Lung* 185: 249-255.

Mochalkin, N.I..(1970). Ascorbic acid in the complex therapy of acute pneumonia. *Voenno-Meditsinskii Zhurnal* 9:17-21.

Muhe, L., Degefu, H., Worku, B., Oljira, B., Mulholland, E.K. (1997). Oxygen administration to hypoxic children in Ethiopia: a randomized controlled study comparing complications in use of nasal prongs with nasopharingeal catheters. *Annals of Tropical Paediatrics* 17(3):273–281

Muhe, L., Degefu, H., Worku, B., Oljira, B., Mulholland, E.K. (1998). Comparison of nasal prongs with nasal catheters in the delivery of oxygen to children with hypoxia. *Journal of Tropical Pediatrics* 44(6): 365–368.

Murray, J.L., López, A.D. editors (1996).. The global burden of disease. World Health Organization, *Harvard School of Public Health, World Bank.*

National Heart, Lung, and Blood Institute Acute Respiratory Distress Syndrome (ARDS) Clinical Trials Network, Wiedemann, H.P., Wheeler, A.P., Bernard, G.R., Thompson, B.T., Hayden, D., deBoisblanc, B., Connors, A.F. Jr, Hite, R.D., Harabin, A.L.(2006) Comparison of two fluid-management strategies in acute lung injury. *N. E. J. M.* 354:2564-2575.

Nursyam, E.W., Amin, Z., Rumende, C.M. (2006). The effect of vitamin D as supplementary treatment in patients with moderately advanced pulmonary tuberculous lesion. *Acta Med. Indones.* 38: 3-5.

Onyango, F.E., Steinhoff, M.C., Wafula, E.M., Wariua, S., Musia, J., Kitonyi, J. (1993). Hypoxaemia in young Kenyan children with acute lower respiratory infection. *B.M..J* 306: 612-615

Panickar, J. (2008). Best BETs from the Manchester Royal Infirmary. BET 1. Oral steroids are not indicated in bronchiolitis. *Emerg. Med. J.* 12:839-840.

Payne, N.R., Burke, B.A., Day, D.L., Christenson, P.D., Thompson, T.R., Ferrieri, P. (1988). Correlation of clinical and pathologic findings in early onset neonatal group B streptococcal infection with disease severity and prediction of outcome. *Pediatric Infectious Disease Journal* 7(12):836-847.

Prendergast, D. (1927). Oxygen therapy in pneumonia. *The Canadian Medical Association Journal* 8:49-51

Raju, T.N., Langenberg, P.(1993). Pulmonary hemorrhage and exogenous surfactant therapy: a metaanalysis. *J. Pediatr.*123:603-610.

Rauprich, P., Moller, O., Walter, G., Herting, E., Robertson, B.(2000). Influence of modified natural or synthetic surfactant preparations on growth of bacteria causing infections in the neonatal period. *Clinical and Diagnostic Laboratory Immunology* 7:817-822.

Reuland, D.S., Steinhoff, M.C., Gilman, R.H., Bara, M., Olivares, E.G., Jabra, A., Finkelstein, D. (1991). Prevalence and prediction of hypoxemia in children with respiratory infections in the Peruvian Andes. *J Pediatr.* 119(6):900-906

Riquelme, R., Torres, A., El-Ebiary, M., de la Bellacasa, J.P., Estruch, R., Mensa, J., Fernández-Solá, J., Hernández, C., Rodriguez-Roisin, R.(1996). Community-acquired pneumonia*Am. J. Respir. Crit. Care Med.* 154(5):1450-1455.

Rojas-Reyes, M.X., Granados Rugeles, C., Charry-Anzola, L.P. (2009). Oxygen therapy for lower respiratory tract infections in children between 3 months and 15 yars of age. *Cochrane Database of Systematic Reviews*, Issue 1. Art. No.: CD005975. DOI: 10.1002/1465185. CD005975.pub2.

Roberts, K.B.(2001). Fluid and electrolytes: parenteral fluid therapy. *Pediatr. Rev.* 22:380-386.

Rudiger, M., Friedrich, W., Rustow, B., Schmalisch, G., Wauer, R.(2001). Disturbed surface properties in preterm infants with pneumonia. *Biology of the Neonate* 79:73-78.

Sazawal, S., Jalla, S., Mazumder, S., Sinha, A., Black, R.E., Bhan, M.K. (1997). Effect of zinc supplementation of cell-mediated immunity and lymphocyte subsets in preschool children. *Indian Journal of Pediatrics* 34:589-597.

Shankar, A.H., Prasad, A.S.(1998). Zinc and immune function: the biological basis of altered resistance to infection. *Am. J. Clin. Nutr.* 68(Suppl 2):447-463.

Shann, F., Germer, S. (1985). Hyponatremia associated with pneumonia or bacterial meningitis. *Arch. Dis. Child.* 60:963-966.

Shultz, S.M., Hartman, P.M. (2005). George E Holtzapple (1862-1946) and oxygen therapy for lobar pneumonia: the first reported case (1887) and a review of the contemporary literature to 1899. *J.Med.Biogr.* 13(4): 201-6

Singhi, S., Sharma, A., Majumdar, S. (2005). Body water and plasma volume in severe community-acquired pneumonia: implications for fluid therapy. *Ann. Trop. Paediatrics* 25:243-252.

Smith, A.H. (1870). Oxygen gas as a remedy in disease. *Advertising Pamphlet.* D.Appleton & Company; New York, 56 pages

Smyth, A., Carty, H., Hart, C.A. (1998). Clinical predictors of hypoxaemia in children with pneumonia. *Ann Trop Paediatr* 18: 31–40

Soll, R.F.(1999). Multiple versus single dose natural surfactant extract for severe neonatal respiratory distress syndrome. *Cochrane Database of Systematic Reviews*, Issue 2.

Stadie, W.C. (1919). The oxygen of the arterial and venous blood in pneumonia and its relation to cyanosis. *J. Exp. Med.* 30: 215-240

Talati, A.J., Crouse, D.T., English, B.K., Newman, C., Harrison, L., Meals, E. (2001). Immunomodulation by exogenous surfactant: effect on TNF-alpha secretion and luminol-enhanced chemiluminescence activity by murine macrophages stimulated with group B streptococci. *Microbes and infection / Institut Pasteur* 3:267-273.

Theodoratou, E.,Al-Jilaihawi, S.,http://ije.oxfordjournals.org/content/39/suppl_1/i155.abstract - aff-1 Woodwart, S., Ferguson, J., Jhass, A., Balliet, M., Kolcic, I., Sadruddin, S., Duke, T., Rudan, I., Campbell, H. (2010). The effect of case management on childhood pneumonia mortality in developing countries. *Int. J. of Epidemiol.* 39: 155-171.

Usen, S., Weber, M., Mulholland, K., Jaffar, S., Oparaugo, A., Omosigho, C., Adegbola, R., Greenwood, B. (1999). Clinical predictors of hypoxaemia in Gambian children with acute lower respiratory tract infection: prospective cohort study. *B.M.J.* 9; 318 (7176):86-91

Valentiner-Branth, P., Shrestha, P.S., Chandyo, R.K., Mathisen, M., Basnet, S., Nita Bhandari, N., Adhikari, R.K., Sommerfelt, H., Strand, T.A. (2010). A randomized controlled trial of the effect of zinc as adjuvant therapy in children 2–35 mo of age with severe or nonsevere pneumonia in Bhaktapur, Nepal. *Am. J. Clin. Nutr.* 91:1667–1674.

Van Woensel, J.B.M., Van Alderen, W.M.C., De Weerd, W., Jansen, N.J.G., Van Gestel, J.P.J., Markhorst, D.G., Van Vught, A.J., Bos, A.P., Kimpen, J.L.L. (2003).

Dexamethasone for treatment of patients mechanically ventilated for lower respiratory tract infection caused by respiratory syncytial virus. *Thorax* 58: 383-387.

Ventre K, Haroon M, Davison C. Surfactant therapy *Cochrane Database Syst Rev*. 2006 Jul 19;3:CD005150.

Von Vigier, R.O., Colombo, S.M., Stoffel, P.B., Meregalli, P., Truttmann, A.C., Bianchetti, M.G. (2001). Circulating sodium in acute meningitis. *American Journal of Nephrology* 21:87-90.

Wang, T.T., Nestel, F.P., Bourdeau, V., Nagai, Y., Wang, Q., Liao, J., Tavera-Mendoza, L., Lin, R., Hanrahan, J.H., Mader, S., White, J.H. (2004). Cutting edge: 1,25-dihydroxyvitamin D3 is a direct inducer of antimicrobial peptide gene expression. *J. Immunol.* 173: 2909-2912.

Weber, M., Palmer, A., Oparaugo, A., Muholland, K. (1995). Comparison of nasal prongs and nasopharyngeal catheter for the delivery of oxygen in children with hypoxemia because a lower respiratory tract infection. *J. Pediatr.*127: 378–383

Wejse, C., Gomes, V.F., Rabna, P., Gustafson, P., Aaby, P., Lisse, I.M,, Andersen, P.L., Glerup, H., Sodemann, M. (2009).Vitamin D as Supplementary Treatment for Tuberculosis.A Double-blind, Randomized, Placebo-controlled Trial. *Am. J. Resp. Crit. Care Med.* 179: 843-850.

WHO. (1993) .Oxygen Therapy for Acute Respiratory Infections in Young Children in Developing Countries. Programme for the control of acute respiratory tract infections. *World Health Organization publications*. Available at: http://www.who.int/child-adolescent-health/New_Publications/CHILD_HEALTH/ WHO_ARI_93.28.htm.

WHO. (2005). Cough or Difficult Breathing. Pocketbook of Hospital Care for Children: Guidelines for the Management of Common Illnesses with Limited Resources. *World Health Organization publications*: 69–108

WHO. (2007). Global Action Plan for the Prevention and Control of Pneumonia (GAPP). Raport of Informal Consultation. *World Health Organization publications*. Available at: http://whqlibdoc.who.int/publications/2008/9789241596336_eng.pdf

W H O.(1990). Acute respiratory infections in children: case management in small hospitals in developing countries. *Programme for the control of acute respiratory infections* 5:1-4.

Wu, T., Ni, J., Wei, J.(2005).Vitamin A for non-measles pneumonia in children. *Cochrane Database of Systematic Reviews*, Issue 3. Art. No.: CD003700. DOI: 10.1002/ 14651858.CD003700.pub2.

Yang, M., Yuping, Y., Yin, X., Wang, B.Y., Wu, T., Liu, G.J., Dong, B.R. (2010). Chest physiotherapy for pneumonia in adults. *Cochrane Database of Systematic Reviews*, Issue 2. Art. No.: CD006338. DOI: 10.1002/14651858.CD006338.pub2.

Yesudian, P.D., Berry, J.L., Wiles, S., Hoyle, S., Young, D.B., Haylett, K., Rhodes, L.El, Davies, P. (2008). The effect of ultraviolet B-induced vitamin D levels on host resistance in Mycobacterium tuberculosis: a pilot study in immigrant Asian adults living in the United Kingdom. *Photodermatology, Photoimmunology&Photomedicine* 24: 97-98.

Zasloff, M. (2006). Fighting infections with vitamin D. *Nat. Med.* 12: 388-390.

In: Pneumonia: Symptoms, Diagnosis and Treatment
Editors: M. L. Suarez and S. M. Ortega, pp. 63-94
ISBN: 978-1-61209-685-8

Chapter III

Quality Improvement in the Nosocomial Pneumonia Surveillance and Prevention in PICU and NICU

***P. A. Fuster-Jorge*[*1,4], *A. Montesdeoca-Melián*[1,4], *M. Mateos-Durán*[1], *M. J. Ramos-Real*[2], *V. Ramos-Martín*[1], *M. B. Castro-Hernández*[2] *and M. R. Montes de Oca-Afonso*[3]**

[1]Department of Pediatric, Neonatology Section, Pediatric and Neonatology Intensive Care Units
[2]Department of Microbiology and Preventive Medicine, of Canary University Hospital
[3]Ofra Medical Emergency Unit, Canary Health Service
[4]Medicine School of La Laguna University, Santa Cruz de Tenerife, Canary Islands, Spain

Abstract

Ventilator associated pneumonia (VAP), the second most common hospital-acquired infection among pediatric and neonatal intensive care unit (PICU and NICU) patients, is defined as the pneumonia that develops later than or at 48 hours after the patient has been placed on mechanical ventilation. In spite of the fact that its incidence is higher in adult patient's intensive care unit, VAP is associated with increased morbidity, length of PICU and NICU stay, antibiotic use and costs also in pediatric population. The lack of a gold standard for the diagnosis of VAP makes an interpretation of the literature complex, and differences in the incidence of VAP occur as a result of the definitions used and people doing the surveillance. As in other hospitals, in our experience the incidence of VAP seemed increase after the implementation of a VAP surveillance program. We have

*1st Author´s post Brit and mail AM: Pedro A. Fuster-Jorge, MD, PhD, Professor Am and Medical Researcher. Hospital Universitario de Canarias; Facultad de Medicina de la Universidad de La Laguna. Ofra s/n, La Cuesta-La Laguna, 38320 Santa Cruz de Tenerife, España. pefuster@ull.es

measured in terms of quality the impact of a specific program of prevention and surveillance of VAP in pediatric population, in a patient-centred model of healthcare assistance. Since 2000 to 2004 VAP represented the 8.66% of all hospital-acquired infections in our PICU. Gram-negative bacilli represented the most of isolates (*Escherichia coli and Pseudomonas aeruginosa*). The medium values of our PICU indexes were 5.52 for the Physiologic Stability Index (PSI), 5.9 for the Pediatric Risk of Mortality Score (PRISM) and 13 (class II) for the Therapeutic Intervention Scoring System (TISS). In NICU data we found 7.50 VAP per thousand days of mechanical ventilation, with very-low-birth-weight infants suffering the highest incidence rate. The nosocomial infection preventive measures, principally the hand hygiene of the health-care personnel and visitors, the correct asepsis before invasive procedures, the adequacy of antibiotics policy, and the correct nutrition of our children have demonstrated to reduce the risk of suffering a hospital-acquired infection even in 50%.

1. Introduction: Ebqi in Canary University´s Hospital; the PICU and NICU; Nosocomial Infection Repercussion in the Intensive Care Units

The Canary University Hospital (HUC) is a healthcare, teaching and research tertiary reference center, located in the Northern Area of the Tenerife Island and belonging to the public hospital network of the Canary Islands in Spain. It has 665 beds and provides medical coverage to refer a general population of children with an average rate of 19.7% and a population aged <15 years of 66.986 children [1].

In HUC many years ago we began the policy of functional standards, proposed in the U.S. since 1951 by The Joint Commission [2], to improve the quality and safety of patient-centered care. Also, in our Neonatology Section, encompassing the pediatric intensive care (PICU) and neonatal (NICU) units, we began this new line of work. Since then, we have developed a comprehensive and progressive master plan with specific strategies and policies for processes that we consider most at risk, focusing on our NICU and PICU in developing not only the patient but also in their family. Even today, we are improve a lot, we are constantly learning, innovating and we know that we have a long way to go to move closer to excellence.

To ensure that each patient receives the best feature set to achieve an optimal process, to achieve the best possible results with minimal iatrogenic (safety) and the highest satisfaction, where the analysis of economic costs should also be able (efficiency and adequacy economic), defined according to the World Health Organization-WHO [3] the overall quality of the institutions, services and health units. All this is included in the organization of healthcare providers in a quality management system, comprehensive processes that will be compared with a model of excellence based on the best available evidence-EBQI (Evidence-Based Quality Improvement) and patient-led.

The Intensive care medicine was born U.S. in the decade of the 60s in response to social and welfare needs of reducing mortality and the number and importance of disability that originated, and it is still produced at present, critical situations potentially reversible. To this end the intensive care units (ICU) were created in specific areas of hospitals, in order to focus on these human and technical resources required to ensure top-quality care, effective and efficient. Also in the early 60s the first PICU was created in parallel with the tremendous growth experienced in those years in the field of surgery and other pediatric specialties; the pediatric intensive care constitutes a specific area of knowledge of national and international prestige and the PICU is the main framework for action, although not the only one, with a very specialized cares for critically ill patients within the pediatric departments and pediatric services. The hospital's NICU are pioneering highly specialized units, which preceded the pediatric units and they served with the highest level of care to babies born very prematurely or whit severe disease; they have also evolved greatly over the past 30 years, gradually implementing the concept of regionalization in perinatal care planning and to introduce the concept of definitive evidence-based medicine; in recent decades there has been an increase in the number of premature births, its causes are multifactorial, affecting socio-economic factors, older age of parents or in vitro fertilization techniques, among others, an in parallel, there has also been a significant increase in the birth rate and survival of premature newborns with very low birth weight- VLBW (<1500 grams), which is generally associated with a very long stay in the NICU, thus consuming 65% of health resources for global neonatology practice [4].

In Europe, pediatric and neonatal intensive care since 1980 had its own society. The current is the European Society of Paediatric and Neonatal Intensive Care-ESPNIC [5], it is an organization dedicated to promote and advance the art and science of pediatric and neonatal intensive care based on evidence, and to meet the needs of this client group so important in the European and international health context. In our country, the Spanish Society of Pediatric Intensive Care-SECIP [6], was founded over 25 years ago within the Spanish Pediatric Association-AEP [7]; the Spanish Society of Neonatology-SEN [8] had its origins in the historical heart of AEP, when the Section of Perinatal Medicine was first created. These two Spanish societies are the nexus of scientific participation and support in the organization of pediatric and neonatal intensive care, and it maintains a close relationship with other companies and networks of intensive care outcome of pediatric and adult, both domestic and international.

To improve the care given in these units, it is necessary to identify risks that have our local population have, controlling the results too. This is essential to establish a registration system that allows self-management results, especially in patients that have more biological and social risk. So, we know our trends in mortality, morbidity and disability among survivors, in short, medium and long term, in various biological areas but particularly in the infants and children neurodevelopment. In addition, our results should be compared with networks with other similar units in their provision of professional human resources, technical and level of care complexity. For many years, this type of network data systems is also available in different countries and communities, some with extensive international involvement. In our PICU and NICU, while continuing to adapt the recommendations, protocols and standards were established by these societies, associations and networks, mainly European and North American.

Nosocomial infections (NI) are associated to healthcare (HAI) and represent a major public health problem in PICU and NICU, by causing high morbidity and mortality, a significant increase in hospital stay and generate increased health care costs [9-15]. Therefore, epidemiological surveillance and prevention must be considered fundamental objectives of quality and safety of pediatric and neonatal critical patient care.

In hospitalized adult patients the NI incidence range is 5-10% according to data from the CDC [16]. This incidence is higher in PICU and the prospective European study of PICU reveals an incidence reaching 23.5% [10]. In NICU it is even higher if we take into account the higher risk newborn, the extreme low birth weigh-ELBW (<1000 grams), in who we find an incidence over 40%, both in Europe and U.S. [17,18]. Being aware of their impact, monitoring and control of nosocomial infections have been a priority in our two intensive care units.

Thus, since 2000 in the HUC an Infection Commission, within the Neonatology Section and the Department of Microbiology and Preventive Medicine, conducted surveillance in our PICU and NICU, following the "Specific Program for Surveillance of Nosocomial Infection in Spain" [19], launched by Spanish Society of Preventive Medicine, Public Health and Hygiene. Through surveillance we obtain various indicators, the most interesting being those that relate the days of use of devices (urinary catheter, mechanical ventilation and intravascular devices) with the same associated infections (urinary tract infection, pneumonia and bacteremia). These indicators are also used by the NNIS (National Nosocomial Infections Surveillance System Report) [20], which since 2005 is integrated into the NHSN (National Healthcare Safety Network) [21]. As a result of monitoring, we have obtained a set of indicators that are disseminated to the PICU and NICU staff. From this information it was established a line of action against the nosocomial infection that included preventive guidelines, which have been developed based on the best scientific evidence available for that, such as the CDC in U.S. [9].

2. Quality of Healthcare applied to Picu and Nicu: Influence on the Nosocomial Infection Prevention and Ventilation Associated Pneumonia Model

2.1 The Concept of Quality applied to Health Systems

In recent years there has been a widespread effort by healthcare professionals for the implementation of plans to improve the quality of their services. Following models originally designed for private business, some European Health Systems, among which is the Spanish one, have initiated the implementation of strategies that seek to improve the quality of health services offered to the people. These plans, product of the effort from different categories of professional workers, are trying to homogenize each other, acquiring international certifications, such as provided by organizations as WHO [3], the International Organization for Standardization –ISO [22] or European Foundation for Quality Management-EFQM [23].

This model is planned on a framework that reports an organization of health care providers and their resources under a system of comprehensive quality management and processes to be compared with a standard of excellence based on best available evidence: Evidence-Based Quality Improvement.

The quality of health care can has many different definitions, depending on the point of view (user, healthcare professional or manager, society), but it is clear that there are critical areas requiring specific plans to ensure continuous improvement, including the patient safety. The fight against iatrogenic in nosocomial infection is hard work and very difficult to achieve, which combines a multitude of factors that require a strict control to avoid potential damage for users that may cause serious consequences: sepsis, exposure to toxic drugs, invasive procedures or even death. The intensives care setting has a higher risk, both by the characteristics of the causing microorganisms and by the high infection susceptibility of the patients admitted at these units [24].

2.2 Healthcare Processes Management

In patient and his environment-centered healthcare model, the instruments, space, supplies and professionals are organized to generate added value that accrues to user, his family, the employees and the society; and if possible, this must be evaluated and improved continuously. Process management is the organization of healthcare activity around the user, which is planning the clinical activity and all acts carried out from the center patient to his discharge. In this way the whole process, i.e. the path that follows the patient for the various services, it is structured and defined improving continuity of care. The process is designed identifying the critical stages of care, solving the detected problems, enhancing measurement systems to lower costs and evaluating the results, all these within the cycle of continuous improvement which requires this management concept.

The creation of an interdisciplinary committee, that would include the clinical service manager and representatives of all categories of health workers, it is imperative to define the processes and to start the model (plan-design-implement-evaluate-act). The involvement of all staff in this new way to understand hospital cares is essential for to make properly all work parts within acceptable economical limits [25].

The same kind processes must be represented in flow charts for its easy and quick viewing and understanding, that in the case of the ventilation associated pneumonia (VAP) its scheme is reflected in the figure 1.

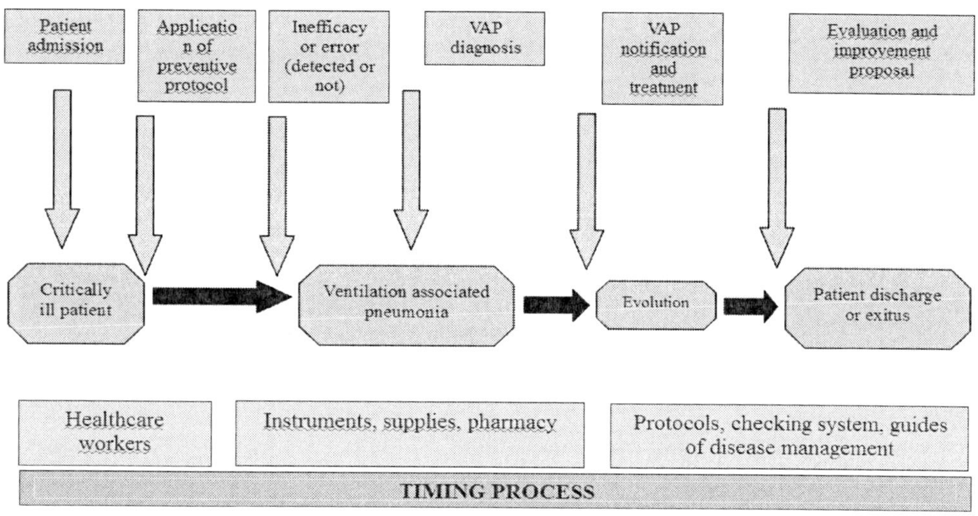

Figure 1. Process scheme VAP (flow chart).

2.3 Nosocomial Infections: Quality and Patient Safety

Two of the primary objectives in this quality concept of healthcare are to ensure patient safety and the efficient use of health resources. Improvement is important across all dimensions of healthcare quality but it is critically important in the area of patient safety. Patients have a reasonable expectation that they will not be harmed because of the healthcare that they receive.

In patient safety and prevention the surveillance and control of nosocomial infections are primary issues to consider, as is reflected in many healths planning documents such as the 2009 National Healthcare Quality Report (NHQR) published by the Agency for Healthcare Research and Quality (AHRQ) of the U.S. Department of Health and Human Services [27].

From that a child comes into contact with the hospital, especially if he needs intensive care, there is an exposure to several risks during the different stages of his stay, these can be initially detectable or not. According of the severity disease and the length of the hospital stay, these risks can be physical, psychological, social, and even behavioral. So this, many hospitals are increasing and promoting prevention strategies, monitoring and reporting the user's adverse events with the idea that "to err is human, what matters is not who did it, but how it has come into, why and how we can improve to avoid in the future" [27]. In order to avoid the errors that impact patient safety, including the nosocomial infections, they first must be detected properly, so they can be deeply analyzed in order to design strategies to prevent them.

Infections associated with healthcare represent an accumulation of iatrogenic damage, both directly (the infection itself and its aftermath) and indirect (derived from the treatments needed to cure the infection). Although from decades have tried to curb their impact on the critically ill, nosocomial infections are still today a serious problem associated with hospital intensive cares, resulting in negligible mortality in both developed and developing countries [24].

In Spain, some studies as SENIC (Study on the Efficacy of Nosocomial Infection Control) have concluded that at least one third of nosocomial infection rates can be reduced only by acting on modifiable factors [28]. This fraction of preventable nosocomial infection is closely related to various aspects of quality of cares, especially with medical instrumentation. Thus, nosocomial infection rates (overall or specific) are universally regarded as a valid indicator of quality outcome of healthcare.

The EPINE (Prevalence Study of Nosocomial Infections in Spanish Hospitals) is the most widespread and used system for the epidemiological assessment of nosocomial infection in Spain [29]. An annual survey of prevalence in acute care medical-surgical hospitals with 100 or more beds is resumed in this study, in recent years involving more than 250 centers and including over 60.000 patients. As stated in the protocol, the study is made with the collection of data from all hospitalized patients for each of which an extensive broad form is filled. The survey is developed over two weeks in the month of May each year. The criteria used to determine the existence of an infection or not, nosocomial or community associated, are the established by the U.S. CDC in 1988, as global reference. The indicators used provide references for management and quality control of multiple organizations and health agencies in Spain [28]. Despite the years since its inception in 1990, the EPINE maintains its full force and has helped many Spanish hospitals to use updated information on the evolution of the prevalence of nosocomial infection. EPINE has led also to a significant awareness in the Spanish health sector on the importance of prevention of nosocomial infections [30].

More precisely, it must be acknowledged that not all nosocomial infections can be addressed in the same way, and there are some whose prevention may be more formalized and thus more homogenized, such as surgical wound infection, and others are not as easily controlled because of mayor complexity. The prevention of surgical wound infections in clean surgery, such validated indicator of quality of care in many centers, is an example of how the implementation of strict protocols that combine pharmacological with various surgical techniques (i.e. Halsted classic principles) can act dramatically in their incidence. However other infections such as ventilator associated pneumonia requires a much deeper approach to be able to lessen their impact on morbidity and mortality of patients admitted to pediatric and neonatal intensive care units [24]. This is because critically ill patients is complex, frequently immunocompromised and subjected to excessive invasiveness and a multitude of acts which pose a potential danger (i.e. broken defense barriers). The control of outbreaks of broad spectrum antibiotic-ressistant microorganisms living in these units is another example of the difficulty to get the goal of nosocomial infection prevention [31].

Invasive mechanical ventilation (conventional or high frequency oscillatory modalities) represents today a fundamental tool for optimal management of critically ill pediatric and neonatal patients, they are especially vulnerable to failure of respiratory function as the beginning of the nosological process that leads to enter a unit intensive care. This means that patients artificially ventilated through an endotracheal tube are exposed to VAP, and they form a high percentage in these units. It is known that the VAP is facilitated greatly by the presence of the endotracheal tube, which facilitates the passage of microorganisms from the oral cavity to the lower respiratory tract, because of it damage the tracheal epithelium, difficult ciliary movement, inhibit the cough reflex and become a place of perfect anchor for the development of bacterial biofilms.

So, the progressive implementation of new non-invasive ventilation techniques implicating to pediatric and neonatal patients has drastically changed the epidemiology of nosocomial pneumonia in PICU and NICU, especially in the very low birth weight premature. It had been detectable in our experience (see section 7).

3. Epidemiology and Pathogenesis of Nosocomial Pneumonia: VAP's impact and Peculiarity in PICU and NICU

Pneumonia is the second most common hospital's nosocomial infection after nosocomial urinary tract infections and is associated with both increases in duration and costs of hospitalization and with excess mortality. Moreover, pneumonia is one of the most commonly reported nosocomial infections among critical care patients, occurring predominantly in those requiring mechanical ventilation [32].

Ventilator-associated pneumonia (VAP) is defined as nosocomial pneumonia in mechanically ventilated patients that was no present at the time of intubation. A nosocomial infection is defined as an infection not present or incubating at the time of PICU or NICU admission, with onset after 48 hours of ICU stay. For diagnosing VAP, the patient is required to have received at least 48 hours of mechanical ventilation and must have two o more abnormal chest radiographs [33].

The epidemiology, pathogenesis, and outcome of VAP well described in adults; few data exist regarding VAP in pediatric patients. The pathogenesis is poorly understood in children, but several prospective cohort studies suggest that aspiration and immunodeficiency are risk factor [34, 35].

In the last decades, the number of premature neonates that need intensive care has increased progressively. Several factors have contributed to increase of the number of neonates with very low birth weight (<1500 grams): the multiple gestations for emergent technologies of in vitro technologies; the development of obstetric technologies for pregnant at high risk; the improvement diagnostic and therapeutic neonatal procedures, as the monitoring, the use of the exogenous surfactant, the ventilation of high frequency, nitric oxide, oxygenation for extracorporeal membrane and the managing of the congenital complex malformations. The patients joined NICU, especially preterm newborns, have a high risk of developing a nosocomial infection. Principal risk factors include the own immunodeficiency of the newborn, gestational age and birth weight; other are the medical treatments, devices and invasive procedures realized during the hospitalization, but these other factors of risk appear only in 70-80 % of the cases of infections in premature newborn [36].

The risk factors for VAP in NICU patients depend on immature immune system. Low birth weight has been shown to be risk factor for the development of nosocomial pneumonia. However, low birth weight may be a marker for an increased duration of mechanical ventilation [31, 32]. Birth weight is one of the more important risk factor to acquire a nosocomial infection in the NICU and for this newborns can be classified in the following categories:

- Newborn with birth weight > 2500 g.
- Newborn with birth weight between 1500-2499 g.
- Newborn with very low birth weight, that defines with a lower weight than 1500 g.
- Newborn with extremely low birth weight, that defines as a lower weight than 1000 g.
- Newborn with a very extremely low birth weight, that is defined as a lower weight than 750 g (this category is considered by some authors) [21, 37].

Also, intrinsic factors can be risk factors to acquire nosocomial infections as immunity or mechanical barriers. The neonates present immunological deficiencies. In preterm newborn several mechanical barriers are upset, for example the skin is thinner. In addition, small grazes in the skin can be a door of entry for powerful pathogenic bacterial or fungi. Another important barrier to avoid infections is the gastrointestinal tract, which can be altered by the use of H2-receptors antagonists, for necrotizing enterocholitis or by surgery [36].

Colonization of the upper respiratory tract with enteric organism plays a major role in the pathophysiology of hospital-acquired pneumonia. After colonization, microorganisms that cause nosocomial pneumonia reach the lower respiratory tract by aspiration. In addition, the stomach also has been considered a reservoir for microorganisms, and bacteria are aspirated into the trachea causing pneumonia. Gram-negative bacilli are the most frequently isolated microorganisms, followed by gram-positive microorganisms [32]

In PICU patients primary bloodstream infection has being associated with the development of VAP, also reintubation, gastric aspiration, mechanical ventilation for > 3 days, chronic obstructive pulmonary disease and positive end-expiratory pressure. Prior antibiotic use, continuous enteral feeding and bronchoscopy have being identified as independent predictors of pediatric VAP [33-35].

Various studies have examined the incidence and prevalence of VAP in NICU and PICU patients. In NNIS (National Nosocomial Infection Surveillance) U.S. hospitals, VAP was the second most common cause of nosocomial infection [20]. The most commonly isolated microorganisms in children hospitals were *Pseudomonas aeruginosa, Staphylococcus aureus* and other gram-negative bacilli. In the study of the European Multicenter Study group found that the incidence of nosocomial infection was 23.6% and the most frequent nosocomial infection was pneumonia (53%), [10, 33, 35].

4. Surveillance and Control of Ventilation associated Pneumonia in PICU and NICU

4.1 Surveillance and Control of the Nosocomial Infection

Surveillance of nosocomial infections provides data useful for identifying infected patients, determining the site of infection, and identifying the factors that contribute to nosocomial infections. When infection problems are recognized, surveillance data allow the hospital to institute appropriate intervention measures and evaluate their efficacy. In addition once can follow the trends of emergent infections that are increasing in incidence, such as pneumonia associated with mechanical ventilation and some times other high risk events as a bacteraemia outbreak. The landmark Study on the Efficacy of Nosocomial Infection Control (SENIC Project) demonstrated that to be effective, nosocomial infection control programs must include the following components: organized surveillance and control activities, an adequate number of trained infection control staff, and a system for reporting the infections to clinics. Thus, the SENIC Project provided the scientific basis for the assertion that surveillance is an essential element of an infection control program [28].

Surveillance is defined as "the ongoing, systematic collection, analysis, and interpretation of health data essential to the planning, implementation, and evaluation of public health practice, closely integrated with the timely dissemination of these data to those who need to know". Population-based surveillance, that is, surveillance of patients with similar risks, requires both a numerator (the infection) and denominator (number of patients or days of exposure to the risk). The essential elements of surveillance are:

- Assess the population.
- Select the outcome (event) or process to survey.
- Choose the surveillance method(s) keeping in mind the need for risk-adjustment of data.

- Monitor for the event or process.
- Apply surveillance definitions during monitoring.
- Calculate rates and analyze surveillance data.
- Report and use surveillance information.

Infection control professionals (ICP) collect data on all sites of nosocomial infection in patients located in ICU and ICU specific denominator data. Site-specific infection rates can be calculated by using the number of patients at risk; total patients-days, and days of indwelling urinary catheterization, central vascular catheter implant, or ventilator support as denominators.

In the NICU ICP collect data on all sites of nosocomial infections in neonatal patients and NICU-specific denominator data. Site-specific infection rates can be calculated by using as denominators the number of patients at risk, total patient-days, use's days of umbilical catheter and/or central line, and days of ventilator assistance for each of four birth-weight categories (≤750, 751-1000, 1001-1500, 1501-2500, ≥2500 g)

Health care-associated infections (HAI) are responsible for significant morbidity and late mortality among neonatal intensive care unit patients. The number of neonatal patients at risk for acquiring nosocomial infections is increasing because of the improved survival of very low birth weight newborns (<1500 g) and their need for invasive monitoring and supportive care. Effective strategies to prevent nosocomial infection must include continuous monitoring and surveillance of infection rates and distribution of pathogens; strategic nursery design and staffing; emphasis on handwashing compliance; minimizing central venous catheter use and contamination, and prudent use of antimicrobial agents. Educational programs and feedback to nursery personnel improve compliance with infection control programs.

The hospital epidemiologist studying the National Healthcare Safety Network (NHSN) [56], recommended the Centers for Disease Control (CDC) [57] definitions for health-care associated infection in June 2008 [38]: CDC/NHSN Surveillance Definition of Health Care–Associated Infection and Criteria for Specific Types of Infections in the Acute Care Setting

4.2 Pneumonia: Definitions and Diagnostic Criteria

Pneumonia (PNEU) is identified by using a combination of radiologic, clinical and laboratory criteria. The following pages outline the various assessment criteria that may be used for meeting the surveillance definition of healthcare-associated pneumonia (table 1, figures 2-3), [38].

Table 1. Pneumonia definitions

Pneumonia PNU1	Clinically defined pneumonia
PNU2	Pneumonia with specific laboratory findings
PNU3	Pneumonia in immunocompromised patient

Report pneumonia that are ventilator-associated (i.e. patient was intubated and ventilated at the time of or within 48 hours before the onset of the event). NOTE: There is no minimum period of time that the ventilator must be in place in order for the PNEU to be considered ventilator-associated.

Location of attribution: The inpatient location where the patient was assigned on the date of the pneumonia event, which is further defined as the date when the first clinical evidence appeared or the date the specimen used to meet the pneumonia criterion was collected, whichever came first. EXAMPLE: Patient is intubated and ventilated in the Operating Room and then is admitted to the PICU. Within 24 hours of admission to the PICU, patient meets criteria for pneumonia. This is reported to NHSN as a VAP for the PICU, because the Operating Room is not an inpatient location and no denominator data are collected there.

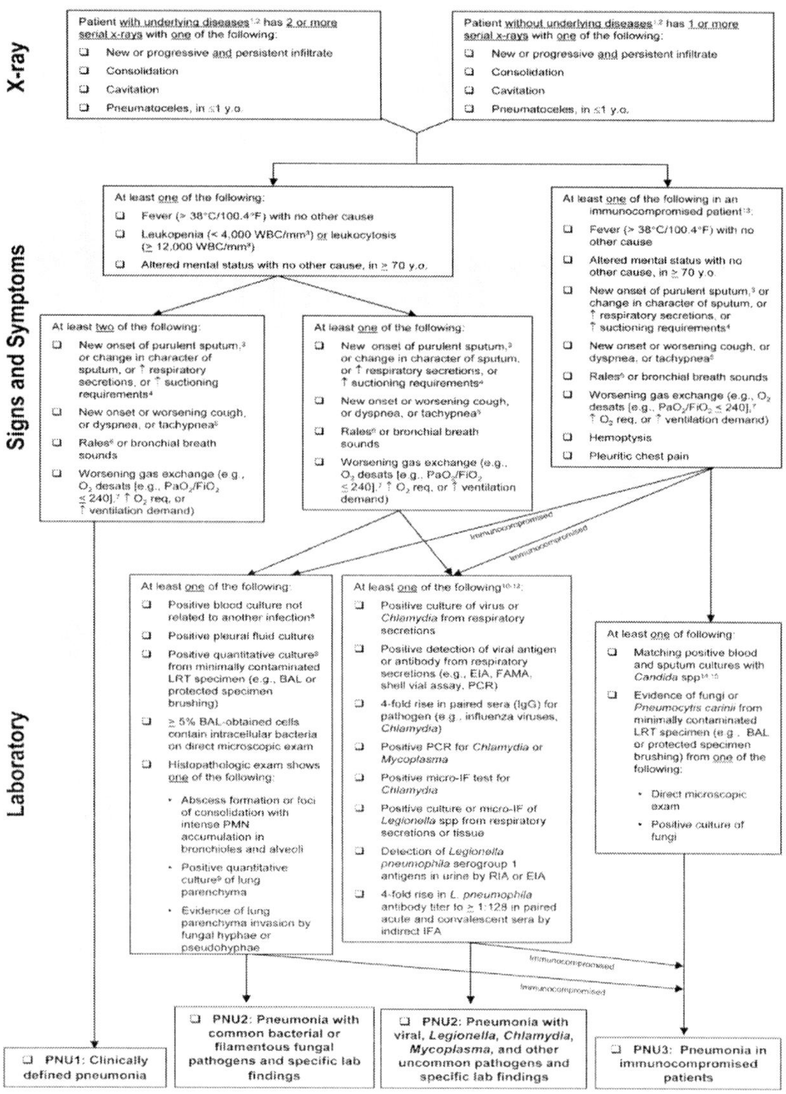

Figure 2. Pneumonia flow diagram.

Ventilator: A device to assist or control respiration continuously, inclusive of the weaning period, through a tracheostomy or by endotracheal intubation. NOTE: Lung expansion devices such as intermittent positive-pressure breathing (IPPB); nasal positive end-expiratory pressure (PEEP); and continuous nasal positive airway pressure (nCPAP or hypoCPAP) are not considered ventilators unless delivered via tracheostomy or endotracheal intubation (i.e. ET-CPAP).

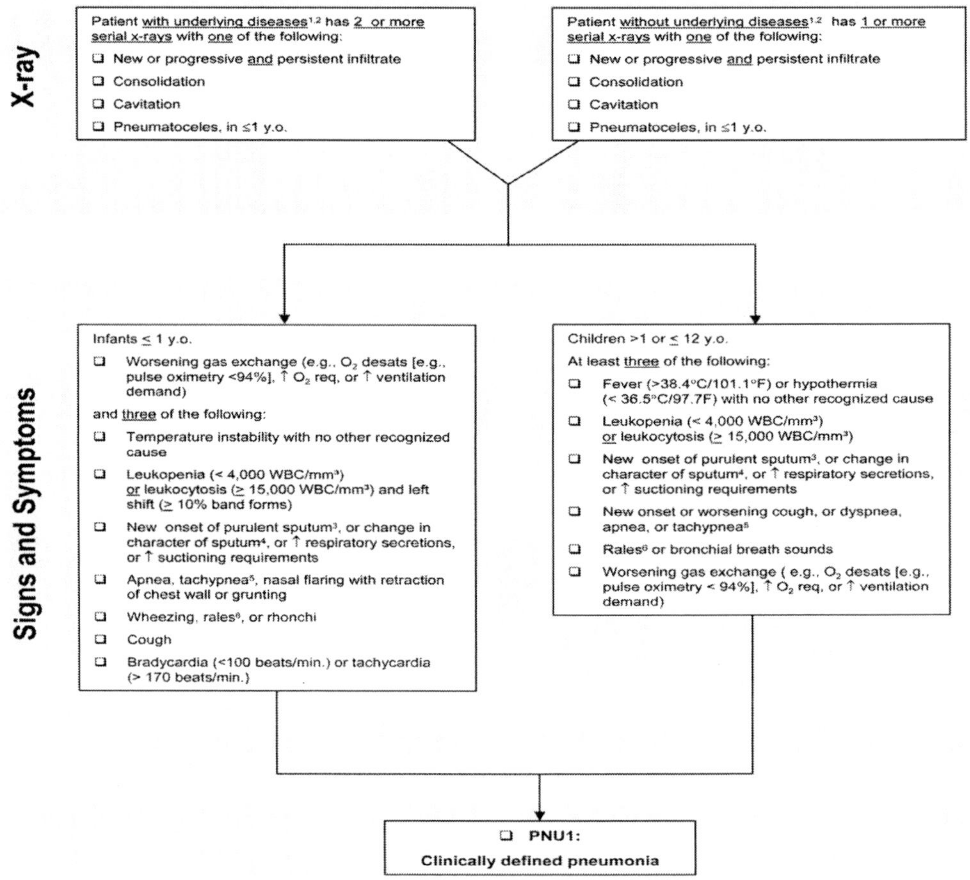

Figure 3. Alternate criteria pneumonia flow diagram for infants and children.

General Comments Applicable to All Pneumonia Specific Site Criteria:

1) Physician's diagnosis of pneumonia alone is not an acceptable criterion for healthcare associated pneumonia.
2) Although specific criteria are included for infants and children, pediatric patients may meet any of the other pneumonia specific site criteria.
3) Ventilator-associated pneumonia (i.e., pneumonia in persons who had a device to assist or control respiration continuously through a tracheostomy or by endotracheal intubation within the 48-hour period before the onset of infection, inclusive of the weaning period) should be so designated when reporting data.

4) When assessing a patient for presence of pneumonia, it is important to distinguish between changes in clinical status due to other conditions such as myocardial infarction, pulmonary embolism, respiratory distress syndrome, atelectasis, malignancy, chronic obstructive pulmonary disease, hyaline membrane disease, bronchopulmonary dysplasia, etc. Also, care must be taken when assessing intubated patients to distinguish between tracheal colonization, upper respiratory tract infections (i.e. tracheobronchitis), and early onset pneumonia. Finally, it should be recognized that it may be difficult to determine healthcare-associated pneumonia in the immunocompromised, elderly, infants or newborns and patients since such conditions may mask typical signs or symptoms associated with pneumonia. Alternate specific criteria for these patients have been included in this definition of healthcare-associated pneumonia.
5) Healthcare-associated pneumonia can be characterized by its onset: early or late. Early onset pneumonia occurs during the first four days of hospitalization and is often caused by *Moraxella catarrhalis, H. influenzae*, and *s. pneumoniae*. Causative agents of late onset pneumonia are frequently gram negative bacilli or *S. aureus*, including methicillin-resistant *S. aureus*. Viruses (i.e. Influenza A and B or Respiratory Syncytial Virus) can cause early and late onset healthcare-associated pneumonia, whereas yeasts, fungi, *Legionella*, and *Pneumocystis jiroveci* are usually pathogens of late onset pneumonia.
6) Pneumonia due to gross aspiration (for example, in the setting of intubation in the emergency room or operating room) is considered healthcare-associated if it meets any specific criteria and was not clearly present or incubating at the time of admission to the hospital.
7) Multiple episodes of healthcare-associated pneumonia may occur in critically ill patients with lengthy hospital stays. When determining whether to report multiple episodes of healthcare associated pneumonia in a single patient, look for evidence of resolution of the initial infection. The addition of or change in pathogen alone is not indicative of a new episode of pneumonia. The combination of new signs and symptoms and radiographic evidence or other diagnostic testing is required.
8) Examples of location of attribution:

- Patient on a ventilator in the SICU is transferred to the surgical ward. Thirty six (36) hours later, the patient meets the criteria for PNEU. This is reported to NHSN as a VAP for the SICU.
- Patient is transferred to the medical ward from the MSICU after having ventilator removed. Within 24 hours, the patient meets criteria for a PNEU. This is reported to NHSN as a VAP for the MSICU.
- Patient on a ventilator is transferred from the medical ward to the coronary care ICU (CCU). After 4 days in the CCU, the patient meets the criteria for a PNEU. This is reported to NHSN as a VAP for the CCU.

9) The following infections are not considered health care associated:

- Infections associated with complications or extensions of infections already present on admission, unless a change in pathogen or symptoms strongly suggests the acquisition of a new infection.
- Infections in infant or newborn that have been acquired transplacentally (i.e. herpes simplex, toxoplasmosis, rubella, cytomegalovirus, or syphilis) and become evident < 48 hours after birth; and reactivation of a latent infection (i.e. herpes zoster [shingles], herpes simplex, syphilis, or tuberculosis).

4.3 Purposes of Infection Surveillance

- Reducing infection rates within a healthcare facility.
- Establishing endemic baseline rates.
- Identifying outbreaks.
- Convincing medical personnel.
- Evaluating control measures.
- Satisfying regulators.
- Defending Malpractice claims.
- Comparing infection rates between hospitals.

5. Antibotic Policy in PICU and NICU: Influence on VAP

5.1 Etiology of VAP

Nosocomial pneumonia is the second most common infection associated to healthcare in the pediatrics and neonatal intensive care units (ICU) after catheter-related bacteremia. In most cases the infection is related to mechanical ventilation for at least 48 hours [39, 40]. The diagnosis and treatment is controversial in relation to the lack of controlled studies of diagnostic and therapeutic strategies in children.

VAP is the most common reason for initiating empirical antibiotic therapy in the ICU; therefore, strategies for the appropriate use of this therapy will have a major impact [33, 35, 41].

It is essential to know the most common cause according to the time of infection, local ecology and patient characteristics (Table 2).

Table 2. VAP etiology

Early bacterial	Late bacterial	Rare bacterial	Nonbacterial
H. influenzae *S. pneumoniae* *MS S. aureus* Sensitive Gram-negative: *E. coli* *P. aeruginosa* *Enterobacter spp* *Klebsiella spp*	As early bacterial plus *E. coli* *P. aeruginosa* *K.pneumoniae* *Enterobacter spp* *Serratia spp* *Proteus mirabilis* *A. baumannii* *S. maltophilia* *B. cepacia* MRSA	*Corynebacterium* *Neisseria spp* *M. catarrhalis* Anaerobics Mycobacteria *L. pneumophila*	Virus: RSV Influenza, Parainfluenza Adenovirus Fungi: *Candida spp* *A. fumigatus* *P. jiroveci*

MRSA: methicillin-resistant Sthaphylococcus aureus. RSV: Respiratory Syncityal Virus.

Prevalent pathogens are different in early (first 4 days after intubation), or late pneumonia. In early pneumonia, microorganisms are common to children's age (*Haemophilus influenzae*, *Streptococcus pneumoniae*), susceptible gram-negative bacilli (*Pseudomonas aeruginosa*, *Escherichia coli*, *Klebsiella pneumoniae*) and methicillin-sensitive *Staphylococcus* aureus (depending on level of ressistance in community related infections by *S. aureus*). Later pneumonia is associated with higher morbidity and mortality. It´s usually related with infections by hospital's environment bacteria and fungi: multi-resistant gram-negative (*Pseudomonas aeruginosa*, *Klebsiella pneumoniae*, *Enterobacter spp*, *Serratia spp*, *Escherichia coli*, *Acinetobacter baumannii*, *Stenotrophomonas maltophilia*, *Burkolderia cepacia*) and methicillin-resistant *Staphylococcus aureus* (MRSA). Those patients with early VAP but with more than four days of hospital staying may have multi-resistant pathogens too, so they will be treated as a late pneumonia. The high prevalence of nosocomial infections by Respiratory Syncytial Virus (RSV) deserves special attention, because RSV outbreak can cause a high mortality in both NICU and PICU and the early RSV detection leads to reduced the antibiotic use [39, 42, 43].

The diagnosis of VAP in newborns is not easy. It should make a distinction between airway colonization and true pneumonia. Therefore the culture results should correlate with respiratory and systemic symptoms as well as radiography and laboratory studies. The causes of neonatal bacterial pneumonia are the same that in neonatal sepsis [44].

5.2 Antibiotic Treatment of VAP

Antibiotic treatment should be initiated early, after getting the samples for culture be . It should be optimal intravenous doses, taking into account the pharmacodynamic profile, combination therapy if resistant microorganisms are suspected or alone if not. The duration of therapy recommended is 7-10 days if clinical response is good. However, in infections caused by *Pseudomonas aeruginosa, Enterobacter spp, Acinetobacter baumannii,* 14-21 days are recommended [40]. In combination therapy with aminoglycosides, they can be suspended at

5th day of treatment in responders. Antibiotherapy will be modified depending the susceptibility of pathogens isolated in cultures (Figure 4), [39].

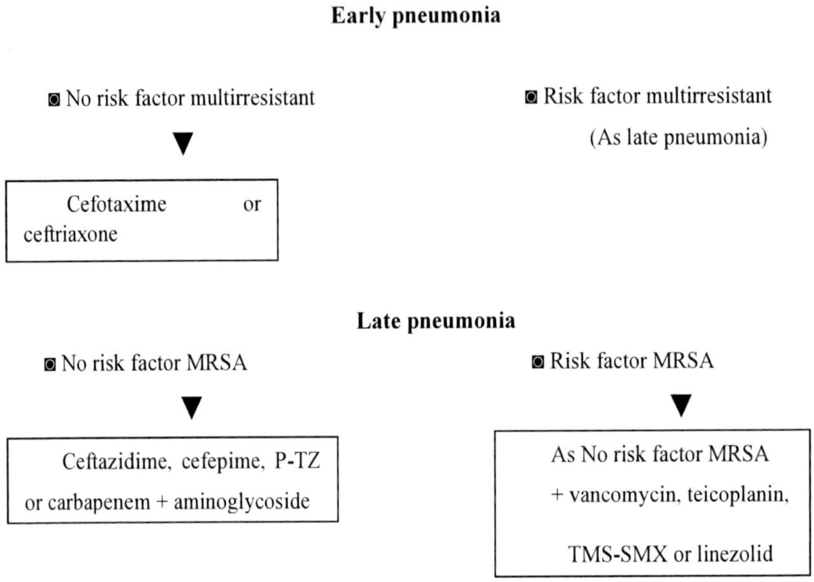

Figure 4. VAP treatment. MRSA: meticillin-resistant Staphylococcus aureus. P-TZ: piperacilin-tazobactam. TMS-SMX: trimethoprim-sulfamethoxazole.

Empirical therapy is essential to assess both the risk factors presented in the patients for multi-resistant microorganism pneumonia and the local epidemiology.

It is recommended as initial empiric therapy, again according to local epidemiology, a third generation cephalosporin (cefotaxime or ceftriaxone). For late VAP, in which is priority to cover multi-resistant germs, the treatment can start with a combination of anti-pseudomonal cephalosporin (ceftazidime or cefepime), carbapenems (meropenem) or beta-lactam antibiotics plus beta-lactamase inhibitor (piperacillin-tazobactam) plus an aminoglycoside (amikacin, gentamicin or tobramicin). Vancomycin, teicoplanin, trimethoprim-sulfamethoxazole or linezolid will be added if MRSA is suspected or probable [39, 43, 45, 46].

The first assessment of therapeutic response must be made within 72 hours after initiation. The appearance of new signs of infection, or worsening should alert that the antibiotics given are not adequate to treat pathogens responsible for infection, assessing the possibility of non-bacterial agents. Cultures must be repeated and changes in the initial antibiotics, increasing the spectrum of coverage should be proposed. In case of good evolution treatment will be continued until the pathogen identification and sensitivity are disposed. If the clinical evolution is worsening although right treatment according to *in vitro* patterns of resistance, it is necessary to determine whether antibiotics given have good tissue penetration, if given the proper dose and interval timer to ensure therapeutic success: peak concentration between 6 and 10 times higher that MIC (minimal inhibitory concentration) in concentration-dependent antibiotics and $t >$ MIC greater than 90% in the time-dependent). It is therefore important to take into account the pharmacokinetics and pharmacodynamics of antimicrobials used [35, 47].

5.3 Influence of Antibiotic Policy of Health Services in the Etiology of VAP

One fact emerging in the last decade worldwide is the increase of resistant strains of pathogenic microorganisms and their possible connection with the massive use of antibiotics. The reduction of the spectrum and the shortening of treatment time are the basis for avoiding the increase of multiresistant bacteria responsible for the increased mortality of this disease. (Table 3) The overuse of third generation cephalosporins has been associated with the emergence of gram-negative β-lactamase-producing extended-spectrum (*Klebsiella spp*, *Escherichia coli*, *Enterobacter cloacae* and *Pseudomonas aeruginosa*) because of their infections no respond to cephalosporins and aminoglycosides, so there is the need for more potent drugs such as carbapenems, with the consequent overgrowth risk of *Acinetobacter spp*, fungi and selection of vancomycin-resistant Enterococci. The occurrence of methicillin-resistant Staphylococcus aureus is a problem that is happened in all hospitals, with a different prevalence by the antibiotics local policy and the percentage of asymptomatic carriers in the patients or health workers. The high incidence of late sepsis by coagulase negative Staphylococcus in neonatal units lead to massive empirical use of glycopeptides, with attendant risks of selecting resistant strains of different species to the same [33, 44, 48-50].

The prescription of antibiotics in critically ill patients do not have to be a routine and defensive event, but a product of a process of reflection which must be taken into account the clinical criteria for suspected infection, the most common cause in each infectious process, the possible resistance patterns of common pathogens, the characteristics of patients and the antimicrobial knowledge.

Table 3. Treatment of high resistance rates microorganisms

	Choise treatment	Alternative treatment
B. fragilis	Metronidazole / amoxicillin-clavulanate	Clindamycin
E.faecalis	Ampicillin / penicillin G + gentamicin	Vancomycin + gentamicin. IMP / MPM /AMP-SB / P-TZ
E.faecium	Vancomycin + gentamicin	Vancomycin + gentamicin+ rifampicin
E.coli	Cefotaxime + gentamicin MPM	Amoxicillin-clavulanate Fluoroquinolone
H.influenzae	Cefotaxime / ceftriaxone Amoxicillin-clavulanate	IMP / MPM / AMP-SB
N.meningitidis	Cefotaxime / ceftriaxone	Penicillin G / quinolone
P.aeruginosa	Ceftazidime / cefepime	Ceftazidime + tobramicina / amikacin
MRSA	Vancomycin	Teicoplanin / TMP-SMX
S.epidermidis	Vancomycin	Vancomycin + rifampicin
S.pneumoniae R	Amoxicillin high doses / Cefotaxime	Cefotaxime + vancomicina / clindamicine
C.albicans	Fluconazole	Liposomial Anphotericin B

Some health services, section and units where be needed the prevention or treatment of infectious patients should have a clear antibiotic policy that must be reflected in a compressive and adapted for himself "guide of antibiotic therapy and prophylaxis". But the prophylactic antibiotic use and antifungal too could be very restrictive because it is one of the principals factors of the higher multi-resistant rates in the pathogenic ecology of the hospitals, to much when it is increasing their assistance level and healthcares complexity, such in the intensive care units.

By that, since 2002 in the HUC we have made a specific protocol for Neonatology Sections that is revised each two years according our clinic and infection surveillance outcomes.

6. Prevention of Vap

Despite advances in supportive care, antimicrobial therapies and mechanical ventilation itself, ventilator-associated pneumonia remains in paediatric and neonatal intensive care. The risk of VAP increases with duration of mechanical ventilation and is expressed as infectious episodes per 1000 ventilator-days.

Several recommendations have been given to decrease VAP. The Centers for Diseases Control and Prevention (CDC) and The Healthcare Infection Control Practices Advisory Committee in their "Guidelines for preventing Health-Care associated Pneumonia, 2003" recommend using orotracheal tubes (instead of nasotracheal tubes) when patients require mechanical ventilation, changing breathing circuits of ventilators only if they malfunction or if they are visibly contaminated and using endotracheal tubes with dorsal lumens to allow respiratory secretions to drain [51]. There are no recommendations for the preferential use of sucralfate, histamine-2 receptors antagonists or antacids for stress bleeding.

Strict infection control procedures as hand hygiene, microbiological surveillance with availability of data on local drug resistant pathogens, monitoring and early removal of invasive devices and protocols for adequate use of antibiotic are crucial in the nosocomial infection prevention and in the VAP too.

Among the literature available in children, some other preventive recommendations have been the following [33, 35, 52-54]:

- Bed's head elevation: the efficacy of semirecumbent position in preventing VAP by decreasing gastroesophageal reflux and aspiration has not been established. Aditionally, size-related factors must be considered in children as elevating the head > 30º is logistically challenging for infants and toddlers.
- In-line suction system: there are currently no CDC recommendations regarding the preferential use of closed or open suction systems for eliminating bronchopulmonary secretions from the endotracheal tube. Also, there are not recommendations regarding the frequency of change for multiuse closed suctioning systems in a single patient. A single study by Cordero et al compared these suction systems in critically ill NICU patients who were alternately assigned to a closed or open suction system: colonization patterns were comparable between groups and there had not any significant differences in the

incidences of VAP and mortality; but 91% of NICU nurses judged the close suction system to be easier to use, less time-consuming and better tolerated though.

- H2 blockers vs. sucralfate: the acidification of gastric contents is thought to decrease upper colonization by potentially pathogenic bacterias. Larger prospective randomized studies on children are needed to asses the impact of stress ulcer prophylaxis on VAP and whether sucralfate has a protective effect compared to other medications that decrease gastric acidity.
- Selective decontamination: This can be done either by using topical antibiotics on the tracheostomy sites to prevent exogenous colonization, or by applying a regimen of topical antibiotics to the oropharynx, and through a nasogastric tube (selective digestive decontamination-SDD) in order to reduce the burden of pathogenic bacterias in aspirated secretions. Also, many investigators have used a short course of intravenous antimicrobial treatment. There is not strong evidence to recommend these practices so far.
- Oral Hygiene: the CDC suggests that healthcare facilities the implementation of a comprehensive oral hygiene for patients in acute-care settings who are at higher risk for health-care associated pneumonia.
- VAP surveillance programmes.
- Educational interventions.

6.1 Evidence-Based Guidelines

The bundle-approach to be implemented has been shown to be successful in reducing VAP and has been used in some U.S. children hospitals such as The Children's Hospital of Boston:

- Avoid or decrease endotracheal intubation, reintubation and duration of mechanical ventilation through protocols to facilitate weaning and promote use of non-invasive ventilation techniques.
- Use of orotracheal and orogastric tubes.
- Avoid heavy sedation and neuromuscular blockade with depression of cough reflex.
- Maintain endotracheal cuff pressures to greater than 20 cm water, except in neonatal and paediatric children under 8 years-old.
- Prevent condensate water in tubing from entering the lower respiratory tract.
- Maintain head of bed elevation at 30° to 45° whenever possible.
- Maintain oral care
- Maintain hand hygiene

In HUC, from 2005 the Infection Commission have make and revised the local "Guidelines for Ventilation Associated Pneumonia Prevention in PICU and NICU" by the collaboration of Microbiology and Preventive Medicine Department and our Neonatology Section and basing in the better available medical evidence. So later in 2008 was made the prevention protocol for other pediatric and adult patients. In the last years we had been implemented each and every one of these preventive cares, principality promoting the hand hygiene, the use of non-invasive ventilation techniques and of closed aspiration system too.

6.2 Future Researches. Future Directions in VAP Prevention

There is scant literature regarding testing the efficacy of head-bed elevation, closed aspiration systems and other measures to prevent aspiration among small children as well as determining the natural history of aerodigestive tract colonization and its relationship to gastric acid in children.

There are some studies about the use of aerosolized antibiotics or altered surface characteristics of the endotracheal tube to prevent bacterial biofilms formation.

7. Our Experience in the Nosocomial Pneumonia Surveillance and Prevention: The Vap Impact in the Picu and Nicu of the Huc and outcomes Improvent

The nosocomial infection (NI) or healthcare associated infection (HAI) has been a critical priority that we controlled and analyzed continuously working with the Department of Microbiology and Preventive Medicine, relating to study the proper use of invasive techniques of greater risk. We prospectively collected the main epidemiological data (number of days of hospitalization, use of intravascular devices, closed urinary catheter and mechanical ventilation) and the occurrence of related nosocomial infections (bacteremia, pneumonia and urinary tract infection).

7.1 In the PICU: Reaching the Quality and Safety Excellence

To be our pediatric intensive care unit a new PICU created since 1997, we prioritize it at the first years. It is an autonomous medical and surgical pediatric intensive care unit of level III-B; it has 4 beds in single box that generates annual revenue of more than 300 patients. During the study period we had an average of 1031 stay days per year, with 65.93% of male patients, a mean age of 3.4 years (SD ± 4.26 and range 0-15). 73% came from the emergency unit, 7% from others areas of pediatric and neonatal hospitalization, 10% from the surgical area and the remaining 10% were outside patients. 46% had respiratory disease, 19% infections, 12% neurological diseases, 10% trauma injuries, 6% cardiovascular diseases and 2% oncohematologic diseases. The incidence of one or more organ failure was 31% (respiratory 39% and cardiovascular 34%) and of multiorgan failure was 13%; with an average severity index of 5.52 (0-26) for the PSI (Physiologic Stability Index) and 5.9 (0 -41) for the PRISM (Pediatric Risk of Mortality Score), which in 26% was >10. Of all patients 39% required only monitoring and conventional treatment, 9% analgesic-sedation for invasive procedures, 64% central vascular catheter, 37% mechanical ventilation, 17% hemodynamic support and 1.8% extrarrenal depurations techniques; with a half therapeutic effort class II = 13 (range 0-50) for TISS (Therapeutic Intervention Scoring System), that also in 26% was >20 (class III-IV), according to the severity of our patients referred to PRISM. Our average stay days was 5.7 (SD ± 8.26), with an occupancy rate of 85% and a rotation rate of 42.8%. The mortality was 3.30% (33% of all deaths where organs donors); the incidence of patients with severe after-effects was 1.5%, 9% of them needed readmissions; and we had a small number of complaints (0-1/year).

During PICU surveillance study conducted from 2000 to 2004 were analyzed a total of 302 patients and NI cumulative incidence (nº nosocomial infections x 100 / nº patients) of 9.76% was found. Predominant localization was as usual the bacteremia that was the 42% of nosocomial infections, with a partial cumulative incidence (PCI) of 4.09%, mainly primary face of intravascular device-related (PCI 2.99%). Respiratory infection was 16.66% of all nosocomial infections with PCI 1.77%; VAP was 8.66% of nosocomial infections with PCI (nº ventilation associated pneumonia x 100 / nº ventilated patients) 0.5% and average rate of days with mechanical ventilation 0.27 days /1000 days of stay; the rate of pneumonia associated to mechanical ventilation in this period was 1.80 and the NHSN average 2.5 [21]. Urinary tract infection associated with the closed urinary catheter was 8.66% with PCI 2.63 ‰, with a utilization rate of 0.37 (closed urinary catheter days/ total stay days).

The principal microorganisms isolated in nosocomial pneumonia and VAP were bacilli Gram negative (46.60%), predominating Escherichia coli and P. aeruginosa, followed by Candida spp (33.30%), predominating Candida parasilopsis, and cocci Gram-positive (20.1%).

VAP had a higher incidence in infants and less age child, critical ill patients, malnourished, immunocompromised, with other severe associated comorbidities and mayor invasive life support.

Tables 4-5 show our results in 2000-2004 for mechanical ventilation associated pneumonia and their invasive ventilation use rates, compared with data published by the NNIS (the National Nosocomial Infections Surveillance System Report), [20].

On the last years after this initial study our PICU VAP outcomes had been the same. These comparative results can be considered very favourable and helped to understand their impact on later to direct time and improvement strategies to reduce infectious morbidity: "Guidelines for the Prevention of Nosocomial Pneumonia in Pediatric and Neonatal Patients" (HUC, 2005); reinforcement of the "Hygiene Program Hands", repeating once or twice a year specific training courses for all the health personnel of neonatology and other pediatric areas too; promoting noninvasive ventilation techniques and early mechanical ventilation winning.

As final conclusion, we believe that the creation of a multidisciplinary working group of infection control, which has involved the Department of Preventive Medicine and our PICU, has facilitated the implementation of effective measures to control and prevent the nosocomial infection. The staff sanitary personal of our units are aware of the need to achieve a steady improvement in safety and quality obtained, among all the nosocomial infection results.

Table 4. Ventilation associated pneumonia the PICU of HUC

Year	Nº of patients with MV	Nº of VAP	Days of MV	HUC VAP rates	NNIS Rates, June 2003				
					Average	25%	50%	75%	90%
2000	10	0	36	0	2.9	0	2.2	4.3	9.0
2001	14	0	66	0					
2002	17	0	113	0					
2003	34	1	253	3.95					
2004	12	0	87	0					
Total	87	1	555	1.77					

VM: mechanical ventilation. NISS: National Nosocomial Infections Surveillance (NNIS) System Report, data summary from January 1992 Through June 2003, issued August 2003. Am J Infect Control 2003; 31:481-98. VAP rate (‰) = number of VAP x 1000 / number of days of mechanical ventlation use.

Table 5. Mechanical ventilation use in the PICU of HUC

Year	Nº of patients with MV	Stay days in hospital	MV days use	Use rate	NNIS rates, June 2003				
					Average	25%	50%	75%	90%
2000	31	235	36	0.15	0.43	0.30	0.39	0.47	0.57
2001	35	301	66	0.22					
2002	65	455	113	0.25					
2003	91	690	253	0.37					
2004	41	373	87	0.23					
Total	263	2054	555	0.27					

MV: mechanical ventilation. NISS: National Nosocomial Infections Surveillance (NNIS) System Report, data summary from January 1992 Through June 2003, issued August 2003. Am J Infect Control 2003; 31:481-98. MV utilization rate = number of MV use days / number of stay days.

7.2 In the NICU: Looking for Reach the Quality and Safety Excellence

In recent decades, several emerging factors such as assisted reproductive techniques, improved obstetric care, the extensive knowledge of physiology and pathophysiology of fetal, perinatal and neonatal cares, and the extraordinary technological advances, diagnosis and treatment in neonatal intensive care have significantly increased the rate of prematurity. These developments have decreased early morbidity but above all have achieved better survival in the premature with a less birth weight (VLBW <1500 grams, ELBW <1000 grams) and gestational age (immature = 28-32 weeks, extreme = <28 weeks). So today the "threshold of viability" is between 400-500 grams natal weight and 22-23 weeks gestational age.

Thus there is a mayor problem for proper respiratory management of this extreme and very less weight premature. In 25-28 weeks gestational age range the best would be to avoid invasive ventilation, oxygen therapy and prolonged endotracheal intubation; ; but in this subpopulation the early and elective administration of surfactant at birth in delivery room is highest recommended for it's tenso-active effect in the immature lung; after this we must to try the subsequent early extubation in the NICU applying a nasal continuous expiratory pressure in the airway (nCPAP), or non invasive ventilation techniques (NIV), and administering caffeine to prevent these reintubation for the frequent premature apnoeas. This strategy has shown a very significant decrease morbidity and mortality, hospital stay and health costs related to the presence of neonatal respiratory distress syndrome (RDS) and the subsequent impact on his mayor respiratory after-effect: the bronchopulmonary dysplasia (BPD) or chronic neonatal lung disease (CLD), [55].

In the last ten years the early nCPAP or noninvasive ventilation techniques from the VLBW newborn birth in the delivery room, that it has been protocol in our hospital since 2003, have meant a change of neonatal cardiopulmonary resuscitation in delivery room and subsequent of respiratory support modality in major world NICU [56, 57]. However, although it's unclear whether this early elective use has a beneficial effect, mainly by avoiding the most common squeal of extreme prematurity the BPD o CLD, or if it causes an increase in the subsequent need for mechanical ventilation and the later pneumothorax incidence, because it delay the classical treatment of RDS, that although it's more invasive, it has proven its effectiveness and efficiency in the last decades [58, 59].

Our experiences is situated in the NICU of HUC, a health level care III-B unit (it's lacking only of ECMO –extracorporeal membrane oxygenation- and cardiac bypass surgery), with 6 open beds and 2 more in an isolation box, that generate more of 300 annual admissions, with an average stay of 7.4 days. Furthermore, we have others two neonatal hospitalization units with 8 medium neonatal cares beds and 10 minimum neonatal cares beds, both with an average of 600 annual admissions more.

We had studied the use of respiratory support techniques and the outcomes in our VLBW newborn (<1500 g) during 2002-2008. We had compared them with the Spanish neonatal network SEN1500 [60] and the international Vermont Oxford Network [61], in which we participated since 2001 and 2005, respectively; and also with the U.S. published outcomes of the NNIS [20] and the SHNS [21]. The reference area of the HUC had an annual average of 3743 live births, with 19198 inpatients and a total of 26198 in the seven years of the study. During this period we had 276 inside VLBW (1.4%), with 117 ELBW (0.6%), and 24 outside VLBW (none were ELBW); so that the total number attended in our NICU were of 300 VLBW. We included only 226 VLBW newborn (81.9%) alive in the HUC with sufficient or uncertain viability (≥23 weeks and 400 grams without malformations non compatible with life, non died in delivery room, without criteria for limitation of treatment) and that were available their parents consent). The average weight was 1146 ± 244 grams and the mean gestational age 295 ± 24 weeks; the 47.8% were male; 19.5% of pregnancies were in vitro fertilization and 35.4% multiple pregnancies; 74.3% were caesarean deliveries; 72.1% received prenatal corticosteroids and 32.3% antibiotics. We collected all the variables into a computerized database, and perform a statistical analysis descriptive and comparative using the SPSS software (+) 15.0. Our main respiratory and infectious outcomes were: in delivery room 78.8% CPR with O2, 58.4% nCPAP, 46% non invasive ventilation by mask (NIV), 31% endotracheal intubation and invasive ventilation and 8% elective surfactant; in NICU 7% early sepsis, 80.5% supplementary oxygen , 74.8% nCPAP or NIV (30.2% exclusive from the delivery room), 66.8% conventional invasive ventilation (44.6% for nCPAP or NIV failure, 53.5% RDS criteria, 9.3% later pneumothorax) and 26.5% high frequency ventilation rescue with a ventilation rate of 0.21 days x 1000 / stay days), 41.1% selective surfactant, 1.3% iNO and 9.3% postnatal corticosteroids to achieve his extubation, 20.8% nosocomial bacteremia and 4.5‰ ventilation-associated pneumonia; at hospital discharge 79.2% home (8.8% BPD -only 2.8% with oxygen-therapy- and 3.1% several retinopathy of prematurity), 3.5% transferred to another hospital (for cardiac surgery) and 17.3% died (1.3% within first 12 hours of life). We found a statistical relationship for the early nCPAP from delivery room or NIV and a less oxygen use ($p < 0.01$), BDP incidence ($p < 0.01$) and severe retinophaty ($p < 0.05$). Besides the exclusive use of non invasive respiratory support helped to achieve faster early and progressive enteral nutrition, a close contact "skin to skin" with their mother and discharge breastfeeding (50%). Outcomes compared with VON and SEN1500 observed: less intubation and early surfactant in delivery room, but more nCPAP or NIV; less oxygen, more nCPAP and NIV, lower incidence of RSD, BPD and severe ROP in the NICU and at discharge, although a higher incidence of later pneumothorax by invasive ventilation, early sepsis and nosocomial bacteremia, while those the VAP and the use invasive ventilation use rates remained adequate, lower length of stay, average weight and home oxygen-therapy. So the early use of non invasive respiratory support had evident benefits but at the same time we should better select the patients that early need mechanical ventilation and surfactant. In 2009 the corrective actions have improved achieving similar or even superior results to those obtained by the VON.

In the 2008-2009 NICU surveillance of nosocomial infections by Microbiology and Preventive Medicine Department, were found 44.30% and 43% respectively. The pneumonia PCI were 3.80% and 10.50%. The isolated microorganisms were, P. *aeruginosa*, Stenotrophomonas maltophilia, *Klebsiella pneumoniae*, *Klebsiella oxytoca* and *Enterobacter cloacae*; with only one case of RSV pneumonia in 2009.

In 2008, newborns with mechanical ventilation were 47 with an average of 7.02 days (SD ± 7.9), VAP PCI 4.26%, DI (density incidence= nº VAP x 1000 / nº stay days) 6.06% and rate 6.06%; in 2009 were 45 with an average of 8.27 days (SD ± 9.12), VAP PCI 8.89%, DI 10.79% and rate 7.50%.

In the NICU, VAP rates (nº of VAP x 1000/ nº of mechanical ventilation days) are stratified according birth-weight and in 2008 they were 0% in <750 g, 15.6% in 751-1000 g, 0‰ in 1001-1500 g, 0‰ in 1501-2500 g and 0‰ in > 2500 g of birth-weight; in 2009 they were 25%, 15.6%, 0%, 8.7% and 0% respectively to this birth-weight ranges. In the study of NHSN rates averages are 3.8‰, 4.9%, 1.4%, 0.0% and 1.2% respectively to the same birth-weight ranges.

So in 2009 we had the highest VAP rate (7.50%) of the last ten years. Previously the second great VAP rate was in 2001-2006 period, but it had decreased in 2007 (5.57%) and

2008 (6.06‰). All HUC rates were higher that the NISS-2003 and NHSN-2006 50Pc (averages), but generally were less that 90Pc. In 2009 VAP were very frequently relationships with the mechanical ventilation use in very critical ill newborn or ELBW with a high incidence of severe congenital malformations, that died around the first life week after completed their diagnosis and had life-support limited. Generally VAP were predominating in more critical and immature newborn, such as the very less birth weight (< 1500 g) and gestational age (< 28 weeks). But in this VLBW newborn we could reduced a 45% the need of intubathion and mechanical ventilation since 2003 with the implementation of early nCPAP use protocol, so that from 2001 to 2009 the VAP rate average was 4.5‰ and mechanical ventilation use rate 0.21, both less 90Pc of NISS-2003.

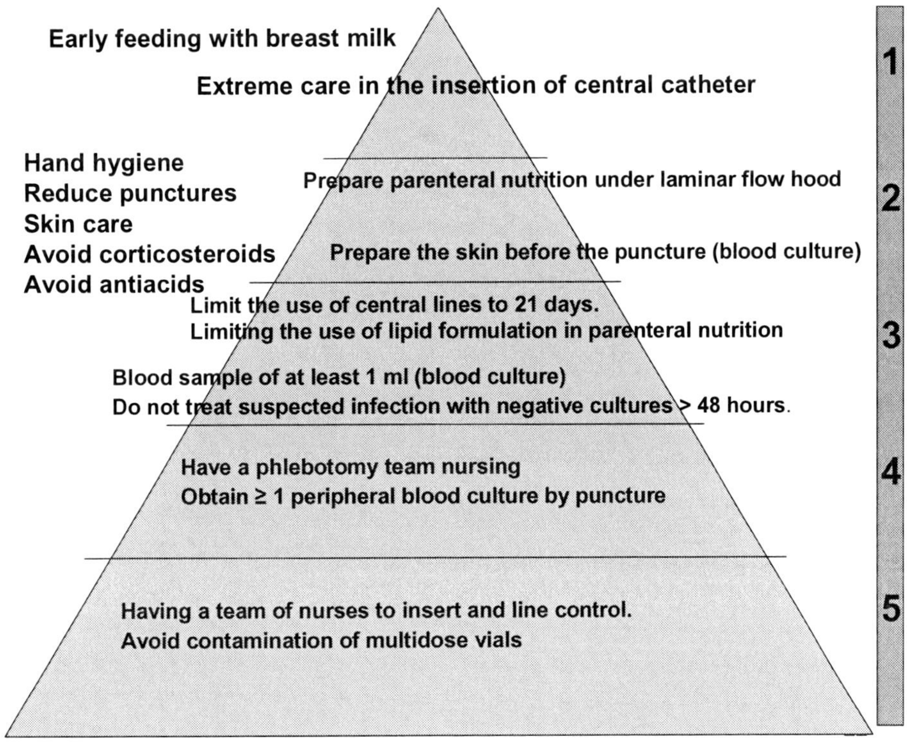

Source (modified): "Evidence- Based Quality Improvement in Neonatal and Perinatal Medicine: The NIC / Q 2000 Experience" (Kilbride et al, 2003). 1-5: Evidence levels.

Figure 4. Potentially beneficial practices (PBP) based on the best evidence available for the prevention of nosocomial infection in the NICU.

In conclusion, our NICU VAP outcomes are very long of the quality excellence but they helped us to understand their great impact on the neonatal HAI and direct and indirect morbimortality. We should improvement too much the actual strategies to reduce NICU VAP ("Guidelines for the Prevention of Nosocomial Pneumonia in Pediatric and Neonatal Patients", HUC, 2005), revising this and NICU antibiotic policy too, reinforcing principally the "Hygiene Program Hands" and the correct asepsis before invasive procedures and the optimal nutrition, promoting noninvasive ventilation techniques and more early mechanical ventilation winning and all other actions that had been demonstrated prevent nosocomial infection in the NICU (figure 4) [55].

Over the years the progressive implementations of these preventive recommendations have to improve our performance, not only in the PICU, but also and simultaneously in the NICU and other neonatal units (medium and minimum cares). So the principal nosocomial infection, the bacteremia has been steadily decreasing, as shown in Figure 5. The nosocomial infection preventive measures, have demonstrated to reduce the risk of suffering a hospital-acquired infection even in 50%.

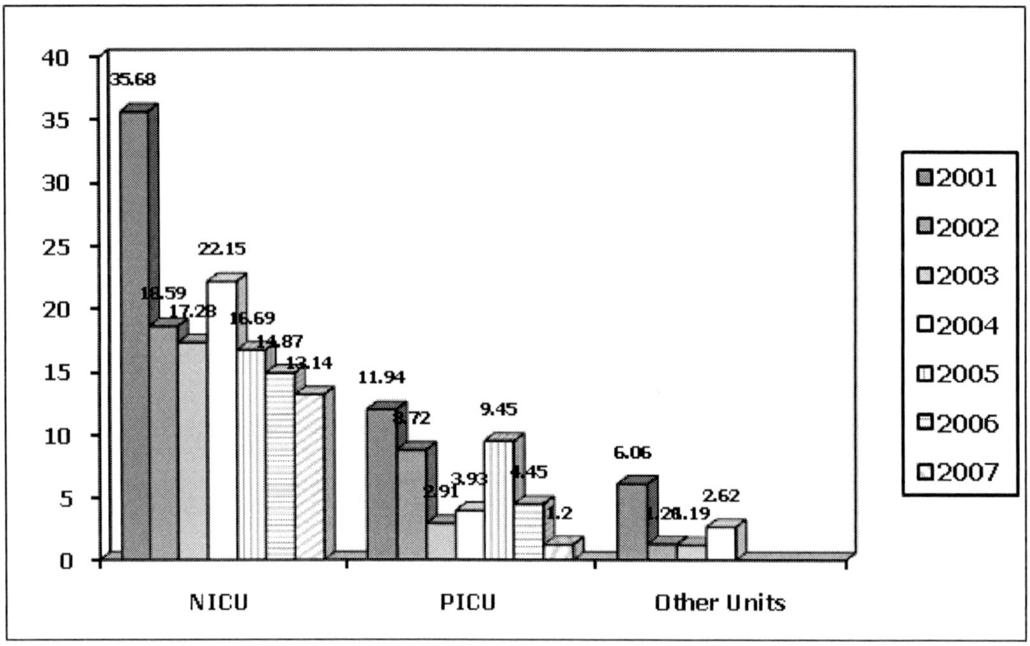

Incidence Density: DI (‰) = nº of bacteremia x 1000 / total stays days.

Figure 5. Nosocomial bacteremia DI in Neonatology Section (HUC 2001-2007).

1st Author Statement

Several parts of ours outcomes studys have been previously reported in the XXII National Congress of the Spanish Society of Pediatric Intensive Cares (SECIP, Tenerife 2005), XXXVII Annual Meeting of the Canary Pediatric Societies (SCP, Fuerteventura 2008) and XXII National Congress of the Spanish Society of Neonatology (SEN, Valencia 2009). Besides part of ours PICU nosocomial infectious outcomes have been previously published in the original paper "Quality control of nosocomial infection in PICU", An Pediatr (Barc), 2008, 69 (1): 39-41 (Copyright An Pediatr and the AEP).

References

[1] ISTAC: Canary Statistical Institute (2010). Retrieved from *http://www2.gobiernodecanarias.org/istac/*

[2] The Joint Commission (September 2010). Retrieved from *http://www.jointcommission.org/GeneralPublic/Complaint/sp_qi_review.htm*

[3] WHO (September 2010): World Health Organization. Retrieved from *http://www.who.int/es/*

[4] Rogowski, J.A. et al (2001). Economic implications of neonatal intensive care unit collaborative quality improvement. *Pediatrics,* Vol. 107, (2001), 23-9.

[5] ESPNIC (September 2010): European Society of Paediatric and Neonatal Intensive Care. Retrieved from http://www.espnic.org/

[6] SECIP (September 2010): Spanish Society of Pediatric Intensive Care. Retrieved from http://secip.blogspot.com/

[7] AEP (September 2010): Spanish Pediatric Association. Retrieved from http://www.aeped.es/

[8] SEN (September 2010): Spanish Sociedad Española de Neonatología. Retrieved from http://www.se-neonatal.es/default_principal.asp?idx=&cidioma=2

[9] CDC (September 2010): Centers for Disease Control and Prevention. Retrieved from http://www.cdc.gov

[10] Raymond, J. & the European Study Group (2000). Nosocomial infections in pediatric patients: an European, multicenter prospective study. *Infect Control Hosp Epidemiol,* Vol. 21, (2000), 260-3.

[11] Lodha, R. et al (2001). Nosocomial infections in pediatric intensive care units. *Indian J Pediatr*, Vol. 68, No. 11, (2001 November), 1063-70.

[12] Stover, B.H. & Pediatric Prevention Network (2001). Nosocomial infection rates in US children's hospitals' neonatal and pediatric intensive care units. *Am J Infect Control*, Vol. 29, No. 3, (2001), 152-7.

[13] Grohskopf, L.A. et al (2002). Pediatric Prevention Network. A national point-prevalence survey of pediatric intensive care unit-acquired infections in the United States. *J Pediatr,* Vol. 140, No. 4, (2002), 432-8.

[14] Urrea, M. et al (2003). Prospective incidence study of nosocomial infections in a pediatric intensive care unit. *Pediatr Infect Dis J*, 22 (6): 490-4.

[15] Edwards, A.M. et al (2005). Attributable Cost of Nosocomial Primary Bloodstream Infection in Pediatric Intensive Care Unit Patients. *Pediatrics*, Vol. 115, (2005), 868-72.

[16] Yokoe, D.S. & Classen, D. (2008). Introduction: improving patient safety-through Infection Control: a new health care imperative. *Infect Control Hosp Epidemiol,* Vol. 29, Suppl, (2008), S3-S11.

[17] Beth, H.S. et al (2001). Nosocomial infection rates in US children´s hospitals neonatal and pediatric intensive care units. *Am J Infect Control*, Vol. 29, (2001), 152-157.

[18] Geffers, C. et al (2008). Incidence of healthcare associated infectios in high-risk neonates: results Fromm the German surveillance system for very-low-birth weight infants. *J Hosp Infect*, Vol. 68, (2008), 214-221.

[19] PREVINE (September 2010): Specific Program Programa for the Surveillance and Control of the Nosocomial Infection in the Spanish Hospitals. Retrieved from *http://*www.mpsp.org/mpsp/Documentos/inf_nosoc/inf_hos.htm

[20] NISS (2003): National Nosocomial Infections Surveillance System (NISS) Report 2003, data summary from January 1992 through June 2003. *AmJ Infect Control*, Vol. 31, No. 9, (June 2003), 481-498.

[21] Edwards, A.M. et al (2007). National Healthcare safety Network (NHSN) Report, data sumary for 2006, issued June 2007. *Am J Infect Contro*l, Vol. 35, No. 5, (June 2007), 290-301.

[22] ISO (September 2010): International Organization for Standardization. Retrieved from *http://www.iso.org/iso/home.html*

[23] EFQM (September 2010): European Foundation for Quality Management. Retrieved *from* http://www.efqm.org/en/

[24] Horan, T.C et al (2008). CDC/NHSN surveillance definition of health care–associated infection and criteria for specific types of infections in the acute care setting. *Am J Infect Control Vol.* 36, No. 5, (2008 June), 309-32.

[25] Institute of Medicine (2001). Crossing the quality chasm: a new health system for the 21st Century. *Washington: National Academy Press;* 2001.

[26] AHRQ (September 2010): Agency for Healthcare Research and Quality. Guide to patient safety indicators. Retriew from *http://www.qualityindicators.ahrq.gov*

[27] Kohn, L. et al (1999). To Err Is Human: Building a Safer Health System. Committee on Quality of Health Care in America. *Institute of Medicine. Washington: National Academy Press; 1999.*

[28] Haley, R.W. (1980). Study of the Efficacy of Nosocomial Infection Control (SENIC Proyect): Summary of Study desing. *Am J Epiidemiol*, Vol. 111, No. 5, (1980 June), 472-485.

[29] EPINE-2010 (March 2010): Study of the Prevalence of the Nocomial Infections in Spanish Hospitals (Protocol). *Spanish Society of Preventive Medicine Public Health and Hygiene.* Retriew from http;/www.vhebron.net/preventiva/epine/protocolo_epine_2010.pdf

[30] Spanish Ministry of Health and Social Policy (2009): *Quality Plan for the National Health System of Spain 2006-2010.* Retriew from http://www.msps.es/organizcion/sns/planCalidadSNS/docs/InformePlanCalidad_ENG.pdf

[31] Schulpen, T. & Lombarts, K. (2007). Quality improvement of paediatric care in the Netherlands. *Arch Dis Child*, Vol. 92, (2007), 633–636.

[32] Yildizdas, D. et al (2002). Occurence of Ventilador-Associated Pneumonia in Mechanically Ventilated Pediatric Intensive Care Patients during stress ulcer prophylaxis with sucralfate, ranitidine and omeprazole. *J Crit Care*, Vol. 17, (2002), 240-245.

[33] Elward, A.M. et al (2002). Ventilator-associated pneumonia in pediatric intensive care unit patients: risk factos and outcomes. *Pediatrics*, Vol. 109, (2002), 758-764.

[34] Almuneef, M. et al (2004). Ventilator-associated pneumonia in pediatric intensive care unit in Saudi Arabia: a 30-month prospective surveillance. *Infect Control Hosp Epidemiol*, Vol. 25, (2004), 753-758.

[35] Foglia, E. et al (2007). Ventilator-Associated pneumonia in Neonatal and Pediatric intensive care unit patients. *Clin Microbiol Rev*, Vol. 20, (2007), 409-425.

[36] Saiman, L. (2003). Preventing infections in the neonatal intensive care unit. In: Wenzel, R.P. *Prevention and Control of Nosocomial Infections.* 14th ed. Philadelphia: LIPPINCOTT WILLIAMS & WILKINS©, 2003: 342-363.

[37] Payne, N.R. et al (2004). Marginal Increase in Cost and Excess Length of Stay Associated With Nosocomial Bloodstream Infections in Surviving Very Low Birth Weight Infants. *Pediatrics,* Vol. 114, (2004), 348-355.

[38] Horan, T.C. et al (June 2008): CDC/NHSN Surveillance Definition of Health Care-Associated Infection and Criteria for Specific Types of Infections in the Acute care Setting. Retrieved from http://www.*cdc.gov/ncidod/dhqp/pdf/nnis/NosInfDefinitions.pdf*

[39] Berrondo, C, & Farias, J.A. (2007). Nosocomial Pneumonia. In: *Critical Child Emergencies and Treatment.* Guide Symptom- Techniques. Intensive Cares. 2th edition. Ed. Ergon. Madrid 2007.

[40] Botrán, M. et al (2010). Nosocomial Infection (II). Other infections. *An Pediatr Contin,* Vol. 8, No. 4, (2010), 174-82.

[41] Bigham, M.T. et al (2009). Ventilator-Associated pneumonia in the pediatric intensive care unit: characterizing the problem and implementing a sustainable solution. *J Pediatr,* Vol. 154, (2009), 582-7.

[42] CDC-NNIS System (2004). National Nosocomial Infections Surveillance (NNIS) system report, data summary from January 1992 through June 2004, issued October 2004. *Am J Infect Control*, Vol. 32, (2004), 470-85.

[43] Del Castillo Martín, F. &, Baquero Atigao, F. *Nosocomial Pneumonia.* In: Ruza, F. Pediatric Intensive Care Manual. 3th ed. Ed. Madrid: NORMA-CAPITEL©, 2003: 1705-1709.

[44] Puopolo, K.M. Bacterial and fungal infection. In: Cloherty, J.P.; Eichenwald, E.C.; Stark A.R.. *Manual of Neonatal Care.* 6th ed. Philadelphia: Wolters Kluwer Health / Lippincott Willians & Wilkins, 2008: 268-295.

[45] Principi, I. & Esposito, S. (2007). Ventilator-associated pneumonia in pediatric intensive care units. *Pediatr Infect Dis J,* Vol. 26, (2007), 841-844.

[46] Hale, K.A. & Isaacs, D. (2006). Antibiotics in childhood pneumonia. *Paediat Resp Rev.* Vol. 7, (2006), 145-151.

[47] Alvarez Lerma, F. & Palomar Martinez, M. (2000). Decalogue of rules for antibiotics use in critical patients. *Med Intensiva*, Vol. 24, (2000), 69-77.

[48] Alvarado Ortega, F. & Herruzo Cabrera, R. Antimicrobial resistant. In: Ruza, F. *Pediatric intensive care manual.* 3th ed. Madrid: NORMA-CAPITEL©, 2003: 1605-1612.

[49] Posfay-Barbe, K.M. et al (2008). Infection control in paediatrics. *Lancet Infect Dis,* Vol. 8, (2008), 19-31.

[50] Riuz López I.K. et al (2007). Resistants in insolated bacterias in patients with nosocomial infections. *Enf Inf Microbial*, Vol. 27, No. 1, (2007), 15-21.

[51] CDC (2004). Centers for Disease Control and Prevention.Guidelines for preventing health-care-associated pneumonia, 2003: recommendations of CDC and the Healthcare Infection Control Practices Advisory Committee. *MMWR* 2004; 53 (No. RR-3).

[52] Srinivasan, R. et al (2009). A prospective study of ventilator-associated pneumonia in children. *Pediatrics*, Vol. 123, (2009), 1108-1115.

[53] Richardson, M. et al (2010). Establishing nurse-led ventilator-associated pneumonia surveillance in paediatric intensive care. *Journal of Hospital Infection*, Vol. 75, (2010), 220-224.

[54] Rotstein, C. et al (2008). Clinical Practice guidelines for hospital-acquired pneumonia and ventilator-associated pneumonia in adults. *Can J Infect Dis Med Microbiol,* Vol. 19, No. 1, (2008), 19-53.

[55] Kilbride, H.W. et al (March 2003). Evaluation and Development of Potentially Better Practices to Prevent Neonatal Nosocomial Bacteraemia. Evidence-Based Quality Improvement in Neonatal and Perinatal Medicine: The NIC/Q 2000 Experience. *Pediatrics, Vol. 111, Suppl.,* (March 2003), e504-e518. Retrieved from http://pediatrics.aappublications.org/content/vol111/issue4/#SUPPLSE1

[56] Burón, E. & Neonatal CPR Group of the Spanish Society of Neonatology (2006). Newborn Resuscitation. *An Esp Pediatr*, Vol. 65, No. 5, (2006), 470-477.

[57] AHA: American Heart Association (2005). Journal of American Heart Association: Neonatal Resuscitation Guidelines. *Circulation*, Vol. 112, (2005), 188-195.

[58] Carlo, W.A. et al (2002). Minimal ventilation to prevent bronchopulmonary dysplasia in extremely-low-birth-weigt infants. *J Pediatr*, Vol. 141, (2002), 370-375.

[59] Vitaly S.H. & Arnold J.H. (2005). Bench-to-bedside review: Ventilator strategies to reduce lung injury: Lessons from pediatric and neonatal intensive care. *Critical Car,* (2005), 177-183.

[60] SEN1500 (September 2010): Spanish Network of neonatal units outcomes and surveillance of very low birth weigh newborn. Retrieved from http://www.se-neonatal.es/default_principal.asp?idx=&cidioma=2

[61] VON (September 2010): International Vermont Oxford Network for improvement the quality and security of the medical assistance to the newborn and families. Retrieved from *http://www.vtoxford.org/*

In: Pneumonia: Symptoms, Diagnosis and Treatment
Editors: M. L. Suarez and S. M. Ortega, pp. 95-119
ISBN: 978-1-61209-685-8

Chapter IV

Ventilator-Associated Pneumonia

***Noyal Mariya Joseph*[1] *and Joshy Maducolil Easow*[2]**
[1]Assistant Professor, Department of Microbiology, Mahatma Gandhi Medical College and Research Institute, Pondicherry, India, noyaljoseph@yahoo.com
[2]Associate Professor, Department of Microbiology, Mahatma Gandhi Medical College and Research Institute, Pondicherry, India, dr.jmeasow@gmail.com

Abstract

Ventilator-associated pneumonia (VAP) is the most frequent intensive care unit (ICU)-acquired infection, occurring in 6 to 52% of patients intubated for more than 48 hours. It is associated with high mortality and morbidity, prolonged lengths of hospitalisation, and also increased cost of health-care. Because of the huge disease burden and the resultant attributable morbidity and mortality, so much importance is given for accurate diagnosis and treatment of this condition. In the critically ill patients on mechanical ventilation, the clinical signs and symptoms of pneumonia are non-specific and varied. Consequently, the diagnosis is difficult and most often delayed. The lack of a "gold standard" for diagnosis further compounds this problem. Although many clinical, radiological, microbiological and histopathological criteria have been suggested by various workers, all of them have certain inherent demerits. The management of patients with VAP is so challenging because of the increased association of multi-drug resistant organisms with this condition. Several treatment strategies and guidelines have been recommended by expert panels for appropriate treatment of these patients without contributing to development of drug resistance. Significant advances have been made in this field over the past few decades, which will reviewed in this chapter to improve our understanding of the symptoms of VAP and help us to accurately diagnosis and treat this condition.

1. Introduction

Ventilator associated pneumonia (VAP) is a frequent complication occurring in 9% to 24% of patients intubated for longer than 48 hours [1,2]. Numerous operational definitions have been proposed over the decades, for diagnosis of VAP. According to the most widely used definition, VAP is defined as pneumonia occurring more than 48 hours after the initiation of endotracheal intubation and mechanical ventilation (MV) [3]. However, in the recent guidelines by the Centers for Disease Control and Prevention (CDC), VAP is defined as pneumonia in persons who had a device to assist or control respiration continuously through a tracheostomy or by endotracheal intubation within the 48-hour period before the onset of infection, inclusive of the weaning period [4]. Moreover, it is said that there is no minimum period of time that the ventilator must be in place in order for the pneumonia to be considered as ventilator-associated [4]. Intubation and mechanical ventilation are associated with 6 to 21 fold increased risk of acquiring pneumonia in hospital settings [5].

VAP is usually classified as either early onset, occurring within the first 4 days of MV or late onset, developing five or more days after initiation of MV. Early-onset VAP usually has a better prognosis as it often less severe and is frequently caused by antibiotic sensitive bacteria. Late-onset VAP is associated with increased morbidity and mortality as it is often caused by multidrug-resistant (MDR) pathogens [6,7].

The clinical diagnosis of VAP is made using the modified clinical pulmonary infection score (CPIS), based on fever, leukocyte count, nature of secretions, oxygenation and the type of radiographic abnormality [3]. But these clinical parameters may be altered even in certain non-infectious conditions.

Many microbiological criteria have been added to improve the specificity of the diagnosis. Quantitative culture of lower respiratory tract samples obtained by bronchoscopic or non-bronchoscopic methods may be useful in the diagnosis of VAP [6]. Endotracheal aspirates are easy to collect and have a high sensitivity [8]. Although an accurate diagnosis of VAP can be made based on histopathological examination of lung tissue obtained by biopsy or at autopsy, it cannot be used as a routine tool for diagnosis because of its invasive nature.

VAP is associated with 20 - 70% mortality [9]. Because of the large disease burden and the resultant attributable morbidity and mortality, there is a great interest in understanding the symptoms and signs of this complication and accurately diagnosing and treating it.

2. Symptoms and Signs of VAP

In the critically ill patients on mechanical ventilation, the clinical symptoms and signs of pneumonia are non-specific and varied. VAP should be suspected in all intubated patients with clinical symptoms and signs of sepsis. The symptoms observed in most patients with VAP are fever, new onset of purulent tracheal secretions, change in character of tracheal secretions, increased respiratory secretions, increased suctioning requirements, new onset or worsening cough, dyspnea and tachypnea [4,10]. In adults >70 years old, altered mental status with no other recognized cause, is a common symptom of VAP [4].

The various systemic signs of VAP are rales or bronchial breath sounds, worsening gas exchange (e.g. O_2 desaturations (e.g., $PaO_2/FiO_2 < 240$), increased oxygen requirements, increased ventilator demand, leukopenia (<4000 WBC/mm^3) or leukocytosis (>12,000 WBC/mm^3) and the presence of a new and/or persistent radiographic infiltrate [4,10]. However, none of these manifestations, alone or in combination, can accurately predict the patients with VAP [11-14].

2.1. Variability of the Symptoms and Signs of VAP

The systemic symptoms and signs of VAP are often non-specific, for instance, fever and leukocytosis can be caused by any condition that releases cytokines like, interleukin-1, interleukin-6, tumor necrosis factor alpha, and gamma interferon [15,16]. Trauma, surgery, deep vein thrombosis, pancreatitis, pulmonary embolism, pulmonary edema, and pulmonary infarction are conditions that are often associated with fever and leukocytosis, as they induce cytokine release as an inflammatory response [15,16]. In a prospective study by Meduri et al, one of these noninfectious conditions were found to be the causes of fever in 24% of the patients [10].

Similarly, production of purulent sputum can be due to tracheobronchitis and does not always indicate pulmonary parenchymal involvement [17]. The presence of aspirated material near the endotracheal tubes in critically ill patients might also increase the amount of secretions even in the absence of VAP [18]. Moreover, the amount of aspirated material is subjective and can vary with patient positioning, gastric emptying, endotracheal tube cuff pressures, and other factors [18].

The presence of asymmetric pulmonary infiltrates on chest radiograph consistent with VAP may be caused by various non-infectious conditions. Atelectasis, emphysema, asymmetric cardio-pulmonary edema, pulmonary contusion, pulmonary hemorrhage, pulmonary embolism, chemical pneumonitis and drug reaction may often show radiographic findings similar to that of VAP, challenging the accurate diagnosis of VAP [15,16,19]. The overall radiographic specificity of a pulmonary opacity consistent with pneumonia is only 27% to 35% [16]. However, studies have shown that certain chest radiograph findings, like progressive rapid cavitation of the pulmonary infiltrate, an air space process abutting a fissure and a single air bronchogram were associated with 96% specificity for diagnosing VAP and therefore can be reliably used. Nevertheless, such specific radiographic abnormalities being infrequent, chest radiographs are primarily helpful in excluding VAP when they are normal [16].

On the other hand, the underlying conditions such as immunosuppression, chronic renal failure, which are frequently present in the critically ill ICU patients, may suppress the systemic symptoms and signs of infection [20].

3. Diagnosis of VAP

The accurate diagnosis of VAP is a definite challenge for the critical care physicians. The interplay of various factors such as the altered immune responses in critically ill patients, presence of underlying conditions, intake of corticosteroids and anti-inflammatory agents, makes the diagnosis of VAP so difficult. The absence of a 'gold standard' for diagnosis of

VAP further compounds this problem [6]. Although many clinical, radiological, microbiological and histopathological criteria have been suggested by various workers, all of them have certain inherent demerits [6].

3.1. Clinical Diagnosis

The clinical assessment of VAP is usually based on presence of fever (temperature >38.3°C), blood leukocytosis (>10,000/ mm^3), or leukopenia (<4,000/ mm^3), purulent tracheal secretions, and the presence of a new and/or persistent radiographic infiltrate on chest X-ray. However, as discussed above, these signs or symptoms individually have limited diagnostic value [21].

Therefore, the clinical diagnosis of VAP was made using a combination of these signs and symptoms. The clinicians routinely suspect VAP when the patient has a new or progressive lung infiltrate plus at least 2 of the following 3 criteria: fever, purulent sputum, or leukocytosis [18,22,23]. According to this approach, respiratory tract secretions cultures were not taken into consideration as they were believed to be nonspecific. Despite being very sensitive, this clinical approach lacks specificity [18]. Studies have shown only in about one third of all patients who meet these criteria pneumonia was confirmed using quantitative culture [15,24]. Fagon et al reported that the clinical diagnosis of VAP was associated with 20–25% false-positive and 30–35% false negative results [20]. Another study involving a series of patients with acute lung injury demonstrated that clinical criteria alone led to an incorrect diagnosis of VAP in 29% of the patients, using postmortem findings as accepted standard [11]. As a result clinicians started using multiple criteria for diagnosing VAP, with emphasize on certain findings over others. One such "weighted" approach developed by Pugin et al in 1991 was the use of clinical pulmonary infection score (CPIS) as a diagnostic tool of VAP [25]. The CPIS was based on 6 clinical assessments, each worth 0–2 points, including: fever, leukocyte count, quantity and purulence of tracheal secretions, oxygenation, type of radiographic abnormality, and results of sputum culture [26]. A modification of CPIS which is widely used for clinical diagnosis of VAP is shown in Table 1 [2].

Table 1. Modified Clinical Pulmonary Infection Score (CPIS)

CPIS points	0	1	2
Temperature (°C)	$\geq$ 36.5and $\leq$ 38.4	$\geq$ 38.5 and $\leq$ 38.9	$\geq$ 39 or $\leq$ 36
Leucocyte count (per mm^3)	4,000 - 11,000	< 4,000 or > 11,000	< 4,000 or > 11,000
Tracheal secretions	Rare	Abundant	Abundant + Purulent
PaO_2/ FiO_2 mm Hg	> 240 or ARDS	-	$\leq$ 240 and no ARDS
Chest radiograph	No infiltrate	Diffuse infiltrate	Localized infiltrate
Culture of tracheal aspirate	Light growth or no growth	Moderate or heavy growth of pathogenic bacteria	Moderate or heavy growth of pathogenic bacteria and presence of the same bacteria in Gram stain

Pugin et al showed that the correlation between the CPIS and the bronchoalveolar lavage (BAL) bacterial index was 0.8, proving that clinical diagnosis can be as accurate as microbiologic diagnosis based on quantitative culture of BAL [26]. In addition, a CPIS > 6 as a clinical definition of VAP, was associated with a high likelihood of pneumonia with a sensitivity of 93% and a specificity of 100% comparing quantitative BAL culture [22]. In a prospective study, a CPIS score of 6 had an odds ratio of pneumonia of 3.0 in comparison to microbiological methods for confirmation of pneumonia. In that study, a score of 6 and no other clinical finding predicted the presence of VAP [27]. In another study, which investigated the role of CPIS in patients with severe brain injury receiving mechanical ventilation, CPIS increased at the day of VAP diagnosis, compared to entry (median, 6.6 ± 1.1 vs 1.5 ± 1.1, $p < 0.001$; sensitivity, 97%; specificity, 100%). Therefore, CPIS could help early detection of patients with VAP [28].

On the other hand, Fartoukh et al found that the CPIS was inaccurate; the mean CPIS at baseline was 6.5 ± 1.3 (range, 3–9) and 5.9 ± 1.7 (range, 3–9), respectively, for the 40 confirmed and the 39 non-confirmed episodes ($p = 0.07$), and only slightly more accurate (sensitivity 60%, specificity 59%) than the clinical prediction [21]. However, they found that incorporating gram stains results into the score was noted to help clinical decision making in patients with clinically suspected pneumonia [21]. Similarly, Timsit et al also reported that the accuracy of clinical diagnosis was improved by providing clinicians the results of direct examination of BAL fluid specimens [29]. A major problem with the CPIS score proposed by Pugin et al is that it requires respiratory tract secretions cultures, thereby delaying the diagnosis by 24–48 hours. In an effort to overcome this problem, Singh et al evaluated the use of a modified CPIS without culture results and found that when the score remained low (≤ 6), pneumonia could be reasonably excluded and empiric antibiotics safely stopped [30].

An important aspect of CPIS, which has been less investigated, is the interobserver reliability. Ambiguities in the scoring system or missing data that were required to calculate the CPIS could result in a large interobserver variability [22]. Nevertheless, Fagon et al found no significant differences in the accuracy of the clinical suspicion of VAP between either individual physicians or physicians grouped by level of training. The likelihood ratios for clinical impression ranged from 2.5 to 5.0 between the worst and the best individual clinicians [18]. Due to its suboptimal specificity, in spite of including gram stains results, the CPIS and its various modifications should be used cautiously in clinical practice, and further refinements are required to improve its value in the management of patients with a clinical suspicion of pneumonia [21].

The Centers for Disease Control (CDC) has recommended the following criteria for clinically defining pneumonia in patients on mechanical ventilation. According to the CDC guidelines, VAP should be suspected in any patient with at least one of the following a) fever (>38°C or >100.4°F) with no other recognized cause, b) leukopenia (<4000 WBC/mm^3) or leukocytosis (>12,000 WBC/mm^3), c) altered mental status with no other recognized cause in adults >70 years old and at least two of the following 1) new onset of purulent sputum, or change in character of sputum, or increased respiratory secretions, or increased suctioning requirements, 2) new onset or worsening cough, or dyspnea, or tachypnea, 3) rales or bronchial breath sounds, 4) worsening gas exchange (e.g. O_2 desaturations (e.g., $PaO_2/FiO_2 \leq 240$), increased oxygen requirements, or increased ventilator demand) [4].

It has been proved by several authors that the clinical approach leads to a large number of patients receiving adequate empiric therapy, while still permitting de-escalation of antibiotic regimens, along with short durations of therapy [22]. Thus, we can safely conclude that the clinical approach to management irrespective of the criteria used will help effective management of VAP, without promoting the unnecessary use of broad-spectrum antimicrobial therapy.

3.2 Microbiological Diagnosis

The microbiological diagnosis of VAP is usually based on direct microscopic examination, qualitative, semi-quantitative and quantitative culture of lower respiratory tract secretions obtained bronchoscopically or non-bronchoscopically.

3.2.1 Quality of Specimens

The quality of lower respiratory secretions is of paramount importance for proper interpretation of both microscopy and culture [31,32]. Improperly collected specimen can lead to false positive and false negative results. There are several recommendations for ensuring proper quality of secretions. The timing of collection of the specimens is very important. The specimen for culture should ideally be collected before starting antibiotics or when there is no change in antibiotic therapy in the past 3 days. The negative predictive value is high (94%) for culture of such appropriately collected specimen [33]. A false-negative rate of 10 to 40% is observed in the presence of prior antibiotic therapy [16]. When collecting BAL, less than 10% return of instilled fluid probably represents inadequate sampling. For the BAL sample to be considered adequate, Baughman et al have suggested that the instilled volume must be 60 ml and the aspirated volume needed to be at least 5 ml with a differential cell count of < 5% epithelial cells [34]. When protected specimen brush (PSB) is used for lower respiratory tract sampling, the brush must be placed into exactly 1 ml of fluid [15,31,35]. When endotracheal secretions are collected they should be aspirated through sterile double lumen catheters with mucus collector to avoid contamination [36]. The catheter should be introduced through the endotracheal tube for at least 24 - 30 cm [37]. After collection of the specimens either bronchoscopically or non-bronchoscopically, the percentages of squamous and bronchial epithelial cells may be used to predict heavy upper-respiratory contamination. The presence of > 1% of epithelial cells in bronchoscopic samples suggests heavy oropharyngeal contamination and such samples should be rejected [32,38]. Similarly, presence of > 10% of epithelial cells in tracheal aspirate also suggests contamination and the sample should be rejected [39]. Barlett's grading system and Murray and Washington's grading system, which were originally devised for assessing the quality of expectorated sputum samples can also be used [40]. The specimens should be processed within 30 min or refrigerated if any further delay is expected to avoid incorrect results.

3.2.2 Microscopy

3.2.2.1 Gram's Stain

The Gram's staining is useful for detecting bacteria and yeasts in the respiratory secretions. The proportion of squamous epithelial or bronchial cells may be used to predict heavy upper respiratory or oropharyngeal contamination [15]. If more than 1% epithelial cells or 10 epithelial cells per low-power field are found, the specimens should be rejected [15,16,31]. When the clinical likelihood of VAP is high, if the specimens show epithelial/ bronchial cells, with few polymorphonuclear cells or when no visible secretions are present, re-sampling should be considered [41]. The number of polymorphonuclear (PMN) leukocytes is generally not predictive of an interpretable specimen in patients with VAP [42]. Nevertheless, in a postmortem study using histopathological evidence of pneumonia as accepted standard, the presence of < 50% neutrophils in BAL fluid had a 100% negative predictive value [43]. The presence of leucocytes was not found to be specific for a positive culture, but in their absence, a positive culture was unlikely as it probably represents inadequate sampling [32,44].

When strict definitional criteria such as presence of bacteria and less than 10 squamous epithelial cells per low-power field are considered, only 15% of endotracheal aspirates (EA) are adequate specimens [42]. A Gram-stained smear of a tracheal aspirate without bacteria or inflammatory cells from a patient whose antibiotic therapy was unaltered in the past 3 days has a negative predictive value of 94% for VAP [33].

Duflo F et al showed that the Gram's stain is highly specific for identifying patients with VAP with 76.2% sensitivity, 100% specificity, 100% positive predictive value, and 75.4% negative predictive value [45]. In this study a good agreement (kappa statistic 0.73; concordance 86.2%) between the final diagnosis and Gram staining was also observed [45]. These results, however had limited accuracy in guiding selection of adequate antibiotic therapy. In the VAP group, the correlation between the Gram's stain and BAL quantitative cultures was complete in 39%, partial in 28%, and absent in 33% [45]. This study suggests that the reliability of Gram staining is variable, dependent on the result of the Gram staining. Actually, Gram-negative bacteria identified by Gram's staining of BAL specimens were highly predictive of Gram-negative cultures, whereas a report of Gram-positive bacteria were poor predictors of the culture results [45]. Hence, Gram's stain is not reliable for the early adaptation of empirical chemotherapy.

In a prospective study for evaluation of Gram's staining, the correlation between the morphology of the microorganisms observed on Gram's staining and the quantitative culture of PSB was found to be less. Gram's staining had 54% sensitivity, 86% specificity, 72% positive predictive value, 74% negative predictive value [46].

The results of Gram stain can be used for modification of empiric therapy. Blot et al proposed using Gram stain findings of EA and of blinded PTC specimens as an aid for therapeutic decision-making in suspected VAP cases. They proposed that when the gram stain from the PTC sample was positive, empiric therapy should be started because of the high specificity of this test, whereas a negative gram stain of EA would suggest withholding therapy because of its high sensitivity [33].

3.2.2.2 Giemsa Staining

Giemsa stain is widely used to determine the percentage of nucleated cells containing intracellular organisms (ICOs) per field. Giemsa staining and its modifications such as Diff-Quik are recommended for evaluation of VAP, as it offers a number of advantages over Gram's staining, including better visualization of host cell morphology, improved detection of bacteria, particularly intracellular bacteria, and detection of some protozoan and fungal pathogens, such as *Histoplasma capsulatum*, *Pneumocystis jirovecii*, *Toxoplasma gondii*, and *Candida* spp. [15,35].

In a study, which prospectively evaluated the diagnostic accuracy of microscopic examination of non-bronchoscopic protected bronchoalveolar mini-lavage (mini-PBAL) fluid in comparison with the results obtained by quantitative cultures, the cutoff point of ≥2% of cells containing ICOs had the highest sensitivity (80%) and specificity (82%), a positive predictive value of 94%, and a negative predictive value of 52%, with an AUC of 0.83 (95% confidence interval [CI], 0.70 to 0.90) [47]. In the absence of antibiotic treatment, the AUC was 0.92 (95% CI, 0.84 to 1.0), with a sensitivity of 88%, specificity of 100%, positive predictive value of 100%, and negative predictive value of 60% in the same study [47]. The direct examination of mini-PBAL fluid was found less accurate when previous antibiotic treatment has been administered. In a similar study, Chastre et al had shown that the presence of ≥ 5% intracellular organisms had a sensitivity, specificity, positive predictive value, and negative predictive value of 91%, 89%, 91%, and 89%, respectively [16].

In the study by Sirvent et al, the accuracy of quantification of ICOs in lavage fluid by May-Grunwald Giemsa stain did not differ from the Gram stain for the diagnosis of VAP [47]. They also observed that detection of ICOs did not influence the management of the patients during the study, or decisions to change or withhold AT. However, they suggested initiation of antibiotic treatment for VAP on detection of≥ 2% of cells with ICOs [47].

In a postmortem study, Chastre et al demonstrated a very high correlation between the percentage of BAL cells containing intracellular bacteria and the total number of bacteria recovered from the corresponding lung samples and with the histologic grades of pneumonia [48]. The morphology of intracellular bacteria observed in BAL fluid preparations obtained from infected lung segments was consistent with the organisms ultimately cultured at high concentrations from lung tissue samples in the same study. Other similar studies also have confirmed the diagnostic value of detecting ICOs using Giemsa stain [29,49,50]. Therefore, Giemsa staining can be considered as a useful aid for selecting an effective antimicrobial treatment before culture results are available.

3.2.3 Culture

The inaccuracy of the clinical approaches for diagnosis of VAP, the impossibility of using such a strategy to avoid over-prescription of antibiotics in the intensive care unit (ICU) and the need to know the etiological agent and its susceptibility pattern has led numerous investigators to postulate "specialized" culture-based methods for diagnosis of VAP. It includes qualitative, semi-quantitative and quantitative cultures of the respiratory secretions obtained bronchoscopically or non-bronchoscopically. These techniques have been evaluated by several workers and each technique was found to have some merits and demerits. Despite their limitations all these techniques have a specific role in the diagnosis of VAP.

3.2.3.1 Qualitative Culture

Qualitative culture is usually performed for endotracheal aspirates. Growth of any microorganism in culture (irrespective of the colony count) is considered as positive [51]. It is widely believed that qualitative culture results may not be very specific and so it cannot be relied on for treatment of VAP patients. Cook et al also showed that qualitative culture of endotracheal aspirate was poorly concordant with cultures that were obtained via invasive quantitative cultures methods [52]. A recent prospective observational study comparing the de-escalation rate between patients undergoing quantitative cultures via BAL and undergoing qualitative endotracheal aspirate showed that the rate of de-escalation was significantly lower in the qualitative endotracheal-aspirate group than in the BAL group [53]. Therefore, it was suggested that use of qualitative culture for deciding on continuation of antibiotic therapy may lead to overtreatment of even patients without VAP and subsequently contribute to development of drug resistance.

Despite this potential limitation and the lack of validated diagnostic standards, qualitative or semi-quantitative cultures of endotracheal aspirates are still widely employed in the management of VAP [51,52,54]. In a recent, randomized controlled trial, which studied 740 critically ill patients with suspected VAP in 28 ICUs across Canada and the United States, the use of qualitative (non-quantitative) culture of endotracheal aspirate to diagnose VAP was associated with clinical outcomes and antibiotic use similar to those that were associated with quantitative culture of the BAL fluid, supporting the use of qualitative culture [55]. In a prospective study involving 219 severely ill patients with a high rate of broad-spectrum antimicrobial use prior to diagnosis of VAP, the sensitivity and the specificity of qualitative cultures of tracheal aspirates was 81% and 23%, respectively, while the sensitivity and the specificity of quantitative culture was 65% and 48%, respectively [51]. As the sensitivity of quantitative cultures of tracheal aspirates was significantly lower than that of qualitative cultures for VAP diagnosis, the use of quantitative culture alone may result in under-diagnosis of VAP, leading to inappropriate changes to antibiotic regimens and, in some cases, antibiotic delay or withdrawal. Therefore, in severely ill patients receiving prior antibiotics quantitative cultures of tracheal aspirates should not replace qualitative cultures for the purpose of confirming a clinical diagnosis of VAP or adjusting antimicrobial therapy. A study by Aydogdu et al also has suggested that surveillance with non-quantitative culture of EA is better than the quantitative EA culture in predicting the development and causative pathogen of VAP in patients who have already been receiving antibiotic therapy [56].

3.2.3.2 Semi-Quantitative Culture

Semi-quantitative cultures are performed by streaking the endotracheal samples onto standard culture media using the four-quadrant streak technique. The cultures are read semi-quantitatively by observing the growth in the four quadrants. The growth is reported as rare (1+), light (2+), moderately numerous (3+), numerous (4+) and heavy growth (5+), which indirectly suggests the approximate number of CFU/ml of the bacteria in the specimen [41,57]. Rare growth refers to growth on the first quadrant with < 10 colonies; Light growth refers to growth of between 10^1 and 10^2 colonies on the first and second quadrants; Moderately numerous growth ($<10^3$) refers to growth of 10^2 colonies in the first and second quadrants, and light growth on the third quadrant; Numerous growth (10^3 to 10^4) refers to heavy growth on the first, second, and third quadrants; Heavy growth (10^5) refers to confluent growth on the first, second, and third quadrants with heavy growth on the fourth quadrant [41]. Some authors use only 4 scales of growth such as rare, light, moderate and heavy [57].

Semi-quantitative cultures of endotracheal aspirate were found to be poorly concordant with quantitative cultures obtained via non-bronchoscopic BAL [57]. In a study involving 256 patients, presence of light growth in semi-quantitative culture of endotracheal aspirate had 63.2% sensitivity and 65.0% specificity [57]. Majority of the isolates missed by semi-quantitative cultures were non-fermenting Gram-negative rods or methicillin-resistant Staphylococcus aureus (MRSA). On the other hand, many non-fermenting Gram-negative rods or MRSA present as colonizers were falsely detected as pathogens by semi-quantitative cultures [57]. So, guiding therapy on the basis of semi-quantitative cultures may result in failure to identify potentially multiple-drug-resistant pathogens, and would also tend to promote excessive antibiotic usage.

In earlier studies using semi-quantitative cultures, presence of "moderate" or "heavy" growth was considered as diagnostic threshold for diagnosing VAP [30,58,59]. However, a recent study suggested use of light growth as diagnostic threshold, as it was found to have a better agreement with quantitative culture. The sensitivity and specificity of the semi-quantitative cultures was also noted to vary remarkably with the diagnostic threshold [57]. Due to the variability in sensitivity and specificity of semi-quantitative endotracheal aspirate cultures and the lack of good scientific data for defining a diagnostic threshold that optimizes outcomes, appropriate antibiotic selection based on these culture methods is problematic.

Currently, there are not many studies evaluating the use of semi-quantitative cultures for diagnosis of VAP. Despite the fact that semi-quantitative cultures are used widely for management of VAP cases, especially in resource poor settings, much work has been done only on quantitative and qualitative (non-quantitative) cultures [30,52,54,57]. Therefore, further studies are needed to optimize the diagnostic threshold of semi-quantitative cultures. If the threshold is optimized, this technique can be considered as a potential alternative for quantitative culture in resource poor settings.

3.2.3.3 Quantitative Culture

Unlike qualitative and semi-quantitative cultures which are usually performed only for endotracheal aspirates, the quantitative culture is done for a wide range of specimens. Initially the quantitative cultures were performed only for specimens collected bronchoscopically such as BAL, protected specimen brush (PSB) and bronchoscopic tracheobronchial secretion (TBS) [60]. Quantitative cultures of samples obtained by BAL and PSB are considered to be the tests that offer the best diagnostic accuracy, but these methods are invasive, expensive, and not uniformly available [61]. In addition, although bronchoscopy has only a low inherent risk even for critically ill patients, it may rarely lead to cardiac arrhythmias, hypoxemia, or bronchospasm [15]. Due to the above mentioned drawbacks of bronchoscopy, non-bronchoscopically collected BAL and EA were also used for quantitative culture, instead of bronchoscopically collected specimens for diagnosis of VAP.

The basis of quantitative culture is that in lower respiratory tract secretions, pathogens are usually present at a concentration of approximately 10^3 to 10^6 CFU/ml, while contaminants are often less than 10^3 to 10^4 CFU/ml [15]. The concentrations mentioned above vary with the site of collection and/or technique of sampling. Quantitative culture was originally standardized by Baselski et al [35]. Quantitative culture is performed by serial dilution of the specimen in 0.9% sterile saline solution. Cultures were reported as colony forming units per milliliter (CFU/ml), after correction for the initial dilution. If the number of CFU/ml is equal to or exceeds the threshold values for the particular technique, a diagnosis of pneumonia is made. Threshold values commonly employed for diagnosing VAP by quantitative cultures are $\geq 10^5$, $\geq 10^4$, and $\geq 10^3$ CFU/ml for EA, bronchoscopic BAL, and PSB, respectively [15,62,63].

Quantitative cultures of deep airway samples were found to have excellent similarities with lung tissue specimens. These cultures can also differentiate colonizers from true pathogens at the recommended thresholds [56]. Quantitative cultures are generally preferred over qualitative culture for making decisions regarding therapy for VAP [64]. However, antibiotic treatment diminishes the accuracy of the quantitative cultures and lowers their sensitivity [65]. Therefore, in patients on antibiotic therapy, the quantitative cultures should be used with caution. To reduce the false negative rate due to antibiotic exposure, samples for quantitative culture should ideally be collected prior to any antibiotic changes in the preceding 24 to 72 h, but if there had been a change in antibiotic therapy the threshold should be lowered [6,56].

3.2.3.3.1 Bronchoscopic Sampling Techniques

Bronchoscopic BAL is usually performed by fiberoptic bronchoscopy after sedation with midazolam plus fentanyl or sodium thiopental. Occasionaly, a short action neuromuscular blocking agent may also be used. Local anesthetics are not routinely used [66]. Meduri and Chastre have standardised and recommended the following technique of performing BAL [67]. Twenty-milliliter saline aliquots are injected each time, for a total of 200 ml (10 aliquots). The selection of the lung segment is usually aided by simple chest radiograph, thoracic computed tomography scan and/or visualization of purulent secretion from a specific segmental bronchus during bronchoscopy. The first 40 ml of fluid obtained during the procedure is referred to as bronchial aliquot, and the last 160 ml as alveolar aliquot [66]. There are several modifications of this technique. Different investigators use varying amounts of saline for instillation and some use the first recovered aliquot for rinsing the working channel of the bronchoscope and reject it to avoid any possible contamination [60].

Bronchoscopic tracheobronchial secretion (TBS) is usually aspirated through the working channel of the bronchoscope before performing BAL. The collected secretions are diluted 1:1 with sterile physiological saline solution and vortex-mixed [60]. In PSB technique, the brush of the PSB is severed aseptically into 1 ml of 0.9% saline solution [60,61].

The various bronchoscopically collected specimens should be transferred to the microbiological laboratory within 45 min and processed immediately. For quantitative analysis, usually the aspirate is either mechanically liquefied and homogenized by vortexing for 1 min with glass beads or mixed with sputolysin and vortexed thoroughly. 100 μl of this sample should be directly added to 9.9 μl of 0.9% sterile saline and serially diluted [61,62].

Chastre et al showed that, BAL had a sensitivity of 91%, a specificity of 78%, a positive predictive value of 83%, and a negative predictive value of 87%, while PSB had a sensitivity of 82%, a specificity of 89%, a positive predictive value of 90%, and a negative predictive value of 89% compared to histopathological findings and quantitative culture of lung tissue [16,31]. Due to their very good sensitivity and specificity, the bronchoscopic techniques are often considered as 'gold standard'.

3.2.3.3.2 Non-Bronchoscopic Sampling Techniques

Blinded, non-bronchoscopic BAL and EA are being increasingly used in intensive care units (ICUs). Many studies have demonstrated that these non-bronchoscopic techniques can be considered as equivalent to bronchoscopic techniques. Moreover, in a study on safety and efficacy of non-bronchoscopic BAL, Kollef et al found that non-bronchoscopic BAL was safely performed by respiratory therapists [68].

For performing non-bronchoscopic BAL, the patient should initially be placed on 100% oxygen. A black line is marked approximately 30 cm from the tip of the outer BAL catheter. The outer and inner BAL catheter should be introduced together through a special adapter placed at the end of the endotracheal tube. The catheter should be passed until this black line reaches the lip. The inner catheter should be advanced distally until it meets resistance or gets wedged. Two aliquots of 30 ml of normal saline should be introduced and aspirated using a hand held syringe [34,69].

The endotracheal aspirate is collected using two catheters wherein a 8 F suction catheter is guided through the lumen of a 14 F suction catheter to serve as a telescoping catheter and is gently introduced through the endotracheal tube for approximately 24 cm. Gentle aspiration is then performed without instilling saline and the catheter is withdrawn from the endotracheal tube. Approximately 2-5 ml of saline is injected into the catheter with a sterile syringe to flush the exudate into a sterile container for collection [8].

Non-bronchoscopic BAL samples and endotracheal aspirate were mechanically liquefied and homogenized by vortexing for 1 min with glass beads [61]. For quantitative analysis, specimens are diluted in a sterile 0.09% saline solution to final concentrations of 10^3 and 10^5 [56].

When postmortem histopathological findings was considered as standard, the quantitative EA culture at a threshold of 10^5 CFU/ ml had 63% sensitivity and 75% specificity, while at a cut off of 10^6 CFU/ ml it was 55% sensitive and 85% specific [16]. Quantitative endotracheal aspirate culture (QEA) also had a high negative predictive value (88.9%), warranting its early use in diagnosis of VAP [37]. In another study, quantitative EA culture was shown to have 88.1% sensitivity, 84.2% specificity, 59.7% positive predictive value and 96.4% negative predictive value [70]. Similarly, studies have shown that non-bronchoscopic BAL has 63 to 100% sensitivity and 66 to 96% specificity [71]. In addition, non-bronchoscopic techniques are cheaper, less time consuming and widely available [26,68]. Therefore, these non-bronchoscopic techniques are considered as acceptable tools for diagnosing VAP [26,57].

3.2.3.3.3 Comparison of Various Sampling Techniques used for Quantitative Culture

In a study comparing the three bronchoscopic methods for quantitative culture, Woske et al found that there was a nearly complete agreement between TBS and BAL (κ index 1.000) and a strong agreement between PSB and BAL (κ index 0.714) [60]. As all the three bronchoscopic methods are having a good correlation, any of these sampling techniques can be reliably used for diagnosis of VAP.

Studies have also shown that non-bronchoscopic techniques are comparable to bronchoscopic BAL. In a study evaluating the usefulness of quantitative EA culture, it was found to correlate significantly with both PSB and BAL quantitative cultures ($r = 0.71$ [$P < 0.001$] and $r = 0.77$ [$P < 0.001$], respectively [61]. Similarly, Kollef et al observed good concordance of quantitative cultures of non-bronchoscopic BAL and protected specimen brush [68]. In another study, comparing the quantitative cultures of blinded bronchial sampling (BBS) and ETA, the agreement between the results of BBS and ETA was 83.3%

[8]. All these studies suggest that the non-bronchoscopic techniques can be useful alternatives for the bronchoscopic techniques in centres lacking bronchoscopy facility.

3.2.3.3.4 Limitations of Quantitative Culture

There is often an unavoidable delay in getting the results of the quantitative cultures [28]. In addition, the quantitative culture results can be influenced by several factors such as the stage of pneumonia, the adequacy of the sample, the operator's skill, method of processing, delay in transport [16]. Prior antibiotic treatment can also result in false negative results unless the threshold for quantitative culture is lowered in such patients [65]. Quantitative cultures can also be associated with false positive results in patients with bronchiolitis and chronic obstructive pulmonary disease, who have high bacterial counts even in the absence of pneumonia [16]. Considering these potential limitations, a quantitative culture that exceeds a threshold value is not always diagnostic of VAP.

3.2.3.3.5 Repeatability of Quantitative Cultures

In a study that prospectively analyzed the repeatability of the BAL the qualitative culture had a repeatability of 95.4%, and the quantitative culture at a threshold of 10^4 CFU/ ml showed a repeatability of 75% [72]. It was observed BAL was a reproducible diagnostic method, especially when bacterial cultures are negative [72].

Similarly, in another study the quantitative culture of EA showed persistence of the pathogenic bacteria at a concentration of $>10^5$ CFU/ml in 82% of the repeat samples, suggesting that QEAs are reproducible and may be useful in diagnosing VAP [62].

3.2.3.4 Role of Serial Culture

Routine QEAs performed twice a week anticipated the etiology of a subsequent pneumonia in 83% cases and aided in prescription of adequate antibiotic therapy in 95% VAP patients ultimately diagnosed by BAL culture [73].

Delclaux et al showed that lower airways colonization is consistently followed by VAP in two thirds (66%) of episodes, supporting the need for serial culture of lower respiratory tract secretions [74]. In a study which prospectively evaluated the role of routine pre-VAP EA cultures in appropriately treating VAP, a pre-VAP EA culture-based strategy was found to appropriately treat 81% patients [75]. In the same study, the positive predictive values of *Pseudomonas aeruginosa*, *Acinetobacter baumannii*, and methicillin-resistant *Staphylococcus aureus* (MRSA) isolated from pre-VAP EA cultures were 88%, 83%, and 100%, respectively [75]. Therefore, it was suggested that whenever one of these pathogens was isolated in routine EA cultures and the patient subsequently develops VAP, appropriate antibiotic for treatment of the pathogen isolated from routine EA culture should be administered [75]. But still the role of serial cultures in predicting the future VAP episodes and its usefulness in guiding antibiotic therapy is controversial as another study has reported that no more than 35% of the VAP pathogens were predicted by routine cultures [76]. Moreover, there is no data to indicate that this approach improves patient survival or reduces ICU/ hospital stay [77].

3.3 Histopathological Examination and Culture of Lung Tissue

Combination of histopathological examination and quantitative culture of lung tissue obtained by biopsy or at autopsy is generally considered the "gold standard" for diagnosis of VAP, as the actual site of infection is examined [16,61]. However, due to its invasive nature, biopsy cannot be performed in all patients suspected to have VAP [61]. On the other hand, histopathological examination and culture of autopsy samples will provide only retrospective (post-mortem) diagnosis and therefore has no diagnostic value.

For ante-mortem diagnosis of VAP, transbronchial biopsy is performed to obtain the lung tissue, but this technique has not been well established [35]. In case of post-mortem biopsy, the lung tissue fragments are obtained at least one hour after death through an intercostal incision extending from the median clavicular line to the median axillary line [66]. The biopsy specimens should be sent in 0.9% saline to the microbiology laboratory for quantitative culture and in 10% formalin to the pathology laboratory for histopathological examination. For quantitative culture of lung tissue the colony count $\geq 10^4$ cfu/ml is commonly used as threshold [66]. Histopathological pneumonia is suspected usually based on the criteria described by Katzenstein and Askin [78]. The presence of VAP is confirmed only when the histopathological findings are in accordance with the quantitative culture results. But, in the patients who were on antibiotic therapy, there may not be agreement between the histopathological findings and quantitative culture of lung tissue. Studies have shown that in the presence of prior antibiotic treatment, many patients with histopathological signs of pneumonia have no or only minimal growth from lung cultures [43,79,80].

The histopathological diagnosis of pneumonia also has certain inherent problems. It is not feasible to routinely perform invasive techniques to obtain lung tissue from all patients suspected to have VAP [47]. Even when the histopathological examination is done, it is very difficult to confirm the presence of pneumonia and the criteria used to define it are not uniform [43,81]. Moreover, in patients with VAP, the lesions of bronchopneumonia may be localised to certain areas of the lungs [79,82]. Therefore, if the lung tissues with the lesions are not sampled, the histopathological diagnosis of pneumonia may be missed. In a study which evaluated the reproducibility of histopathological diagnosis of pneumonia, there was a significant variation of about 18% to 38% in interpretation of the histopathological findings by different pathologists [81].

3.3.1 Challenges in using Histopathological Examination and Culture of Lung Tissue as 'Gold Standard'

In addition to the above mentioned demerits of the histopathological findings and lung tissue cultures, there are certain precautions to be taken while using these methods as 'gold standard' for evaluating other diagnostic techniques of VAP. Based on histopathological examination it will not be possible to distinguish a recent infection from the sequelae of a previous infection [83]. So, when histopathological results are used as standard, we have to ensure that the patient did not have any other lung infection in the recent past. As studies have shown that prior antibiotic therapy can lead to false negative culture reports, while evaluating the accuracy of any technique that uses lung cultures as the 'gold standard', it is necessary to confirm if there was a recent change in antibiotic or addition of new antibiotic. Furthermore, patients included in the postmortem studies may not be truly representative of most patients with VAP and so the evaluation of other diagnostic tools in comparison to these "gold standards" may not be fully justified [16].

4. Epidemiological Investigation of VAP

The epidemiology of VAP is more complex because of the coexistence of epidemic cases due to the ICU strain with unrelated sporadic cases caused by different strains. Use of molecular typing methods is essential to improve the detection of microepidemics amenable to early control. In an epidemiological investigation by Alfieri et al it was shown that the isolates recovered from ventilators, an in-line suction catheter and patients with VAP were the same based on restriction fragment-length polymorphism typing by pulsed-field gel electrophoresis (PFGE) [84]. They have concluded that such molecular typing methods are useful in detecting outbreaks caused by organisms spreading from contaminated equipment or an environmental source [84]. In another similar study, the same strains of *Pseudomonas aeruginosa* and *Acinetobacter baumannii* were isolated from patients with VAP and also from the ICU milieu [85]. In that study PCR-RFLP and antibiogram typing were used to identify the similar strains. In a study concerning nosocomially acquired *Acinetobacter baumannii* infection, ribotyping showed that an epidemic of 11 cases was coexisting with 17 sporadic cases characterized by the diversity of the banding patterns of the isolates [86]. Therefore, the molecular typing methods are essential to confirm if the environmental or the health care worker associated microorganism is responsible for VAP in the ICU patients, so that control measures can be implemented to prevent new cases of VAP.

5. Treatment

The successful treatment of patients with VAP remains a challenge for critical care physicians as it is influenced by diverse factors including lack of definitive diagnosis of VAP, lack of an adequate technique/ facility to directly sample the infection site in the lung, difficulty in differentiating active infection from colonization, and increased occurrence of MDR pathogens [7,15,87].

The American Thoracic Society (ATS) has formulated certain guidelines for management of patients with VAP [6]. Prompt and early administration of antibiotic therapy is very important as a delay in appropriate antibiotic therapy is associated with excess morbidity and mortality [6]. In a prospective study, patients with VAP, who had received inappropriate therapy and those with delayed initiation of appropriate therapy, were observed to have increased CPIS and high mortality rate [88]. Similarly, in another study, VAP patients receiving partially or totally inappropriate therapy were found to have significantly high mortality rate (Relative risk, 2.00; 95% confidence interval, 1.14 to 3.52; *P* 0.0008). Moreover, a delay of more than 2 days in administering the first dose of appropriate antibiotic therapy was observed to significantly prolong the duration of ventilation [89]. Although early appropriate antibiotics improves survival of patients with VAP, the risk of colonization and subsequent superinfection with MDR pathogens warns against the indiscriminate use of empiric broad-spectrum antibiotics in patients without infection [15]. This emphasizes the need to accurately identify the patients with VAP. The initial empiric therapy should be selected based on the presence or absence of risk factors for MDR pathogens such as prolonged hospitalization, admission from a healthcare-related facility, and prior antibiotic therapy. The empirical antibiotic therapy recommended by the ATS is shown in Table 2 [6]. Piperacillin/tazobactam in combination with either aminoglycoside or ciprofloxacin has been recognised as an effective regimen for empiric therapy [90]. A prospective study has documented that an initial empiric therapy with antipseudomonal penicillins plus β-lactamase inhibitor was associated with lower in-hospital mortality. Addition of gentamicin to the above regimen was found to further reduce the mortality [91]. A combination regimen including an antipseudomonal carbapenem or an antipseudomonal cephalosporin with either a fluoroquinolone or an aminoglycoside is a good alternative regimen for empirical therapy [19]. The aminoglycosides have poor lung penetration and so they should not be used as monotherapy [19].

Table 2. Initial Empirical Therapy for VAP

Patients with known risk factors for MDR pathogens	Patients with no risk factors for MDR pathogens
Antipseudomonal cephalosporin (cefepime, ceftazidime) *or* Antipseudomonal carbepenem (imipenem or meropenem) *or* β-Lactam/ β-lactamase inhibitor (piperacillin–tazobactam) *plus* Antipseudomonal fluoroquinolone (ciprofloxacin or levofloxacin) *or* Aminoglycoside (amikacin, gentamicin, or tobramycin) *plus* Linezolid or vancomycin (if risk factors for MRSA are present)	Ceftriaxone *or* Levofloxacin, moxifloxacin, or ciprofloxacin *or* Ampicillin/sulbactam *or* Ertapenem

MDR = Multidrug-resistant
MRSA = Methicillin-resistant *Staphylococcus aureus*

The selection of specific agents should be based on cost, feasibility, availability and knowledge of local microbial flora [6]. Porzecanski et al observed that an approach based on the antibiotic susceptibility pattern of the local hospital or ICU pathogens, has the potential to increase the likelihood of adequate initial antibiotic therapy and therefore can reduce the overall use of antibiotics and the associated selection pressure for MDR bacteria [92]. A different class of antibiotic should be used as empiric therapy for patients who have recently received an antibiotic, as recent therapy predisposes to resistance to that same class of antibiotics increasing the probability of inappropriate therapy. Combination therapy should be employed in patients likely to be infected with MDR pathogens [6]. Whenever a good clinical response with resolution of clinical features of infection is observed, the duration of empiric therapy should be shortened from the traditional 14 to 21 days to about 7 days [6]. A randomized controlled trial proved that an antibiotic discontinuation policy based on clinical evidence of a resolving VAP was associated with a decrease in the overall duration of antibiotic treatment [93]. However, when *P. aeruginosa*, *Acinetobacter* species or other non-fermenters were identified as pathogens prolonged duration of treatment is recommended [6].

5.1 De-Escalation Strategy

De-escalation strategy is a promising approach for effective management of VAP patients without contributing to development of drug resistance [6,87]. According to this approach, the VAP patients are initially treated with broad spectrum antibiotic regimen and later based on the clinical response and culture results the antibiotics are tailored down and unnecessary antibiotics are withdrawn [6,94]. The initial broad spectrum antibiotic coverage ensures early administration of appropriate therapy and reduces the chance of inadequate treatment, while the narrowing of antibiotics based on culture results decreases the risk of development of drug resistance [94].

Though this strategy has been proved to be effective, there is a practical difficulty in treating patients with culture negative BAL despite a high index of clinical suspicion of VAP. Based on a prospective study, Kollef et al suggested that patients with a clinical suspicion of VAP and culture-negative BAL can have empiric antimicrobial therapy safely discontinued within 72 h or in some cases withheld altogether [95]. However, randomized clinical trials involving large number of patients are necessary to establish the safety of employing culture-negative BAL as the primary criterion for the discontinuation of empirical antibiotic treatment, as it is well known that prior antibiotic treatment could result in false negative BAL culture even in patients with VAP.

5.2 Short-Course Therapy

Deciding the appropriate duration of treatment for patients with VAP is a challenge. An unduly prolonged duration of antibiotic treatment may favor development of drug resistance, while a short course of treatment may result in treatment failure or relapse [93]. Despite being fully aware of this problem, most cases of VAP are traditionally treated for a period of 14 – 21 days. But such a prolonged duration of treatment has a certain drawback. Dennesen et al had shown that during the second week of therapy Gram-negative pathogens reemerged and colonized the trachea. They also observed that the colonization subsequently led to recurrence of VAP due to drug resistant strains [96]. This emphasizes the need to have short course of treatment, so that there is no risk of colonization by drug resistant pathogens. In a large randomized trial comparing the short course (8 days) of antibiotic therapy and the traditional 15 days treatment, Chastre et al found that both the courses had similar efficacy, but the longer course of antibiotic therapy was associated with statistically greater emergence of multiply resistant bacteria [97]. Therefore, the short course of treatment was observed to perform better. However, pulmonary infections due to non-fermenting Gram-negative bacilli recurred more frequently with the short course, although in this subpopulation mortality and outcomes were similar regardless of the duration of antibiotic therapy [97]. So, the authors suggested that short-courses are adequate to successfully treat most patients with VAP, but those infected with non-fermenters should be treated for a prolonged duration. Singh et al suggested that the short course of empiric therapy should be used for patients with modified CPIS ≤ 6, while longer duration is needed for those with CPIS > 6 [30].

5.3 Aerosolized Antibiotics

Aerosolization is a way to enhance antibiotic penetration to the lower respiratory tract [6]. Aminoglycosides and polymyxin B (colistin) are the widely used and studied aerosolised antibiotics [6]. In a recent study, use of nebulized colistin was shown to be reasonably efficacious and safe for treatment of MDR *Pseudomonas aeruginosa* and *Acinetobacter baumannii* with an overall clinical and microbiological response rates of 57.1% and 85.7%, respectively [98]. In another prospective randomized trial, the adjunctive use of locally instilled tobramycin with intravenous therapy in the treatment of VAP was shown to achieve a significantly greater microbiologic eradication. However, there was no significant improvement in the clinical outcome compared with placebo [99].

Hamer et al have observed that patients with VAP due to MDR *P. aeruginosa* that was unresponsive to systemic antibiotics, had improved with the addition of aerosolized aminoglycosides or polymyxin B [100]. Therefore, aerosolized antibiotics may be useful to treat microorganisms which are resistant to systemic therapy owing to their high MIC values. However, there is lack of sufficient clinical evidence to support the use of aerosolized antibiotics in established VAP [6,101]. Polymyxin aerosols have been suggested to be useful for prevention of gram-negative bacillary pneumonia [102]. But, its potential to increase the risk of VAP due to MDR pathogens warns against its prophylactic use. The current ATS guidelines does not recommend its routine use in management of VAP patients, however it is suggested that the aerosolised antibiotics may have an adjunctive role [6].

The aerosolized antibiotics have several limitations including high cost, development of antibiotic resistance, inability to treat deep sited infections and serious adverse effects such as bronchospasm and systemic toxicity due to increased absorption of the drugs across inflamed airway [6,101]. Therefore, further studies are needed before recommending their routine use in treating patients with VAP.

References

[1] Morehead, RS; Pinto, SJ. Ventilator-associated pneumonia. Arch Intern Med, 2000,160,1926-36.

[2] Joseph, NM; Sistla, S; Dutta, TK; Badhe, AS; Parija, SC. Ventilator-associated pneumonia in a tertiary care hospital in India: incidence and risk factors. J Infect Dev Ctries,2009,3,771-7.

[3] Davis, KA. Ventilator-associated pneumonia: a review. J Intensive Care Med, 2006,21,211-26.

[4] Centers for Disease Control and Prevention. Ventilator-Associated Pneumonia (VAP) Event. Guidelines and procedures for monitoring VAP. 2009 [cited 2009 Jul 22]. Available from:www.cdc.gov/nhsn/PDFs/pscManual/6pscVAPcurrent .pdf
[5] Weber, DJ; Rutala, WA; Mayhall, CG. Nosocomial respiratory tract infections and Gram negative pneumonia. In: Fishman AP, Elias JA, Fishman JA, Grippi MA, Kaiser LR, Senior RM, editors. Pulmonary disease and disorders. 3rd ed. New York: McGraw-Hill; 1998, 2213-27.
[6] Niederman, MS; Craven, DE. Guidelines for the management of adults with hospital-acquired, ventilator-associated, and healthcare-associated pneumonia. Am J Respir Crit Care Med,2005,171,388-416.
[7] Joseph, NM; Sistla, S; Dutta, TK; Badhe, AS; Rasitha, D; Parija, SC. Ventilator-associated pneumonia in a tertiary care hospital in India: role of multi-drug resistant pathogens. J Infect Dev Ctries,2010,4,218-25.
[8] Rajasekhar, T; Anuradha, K; Suhasini, T; Lakshmi, V. The role of quantitative cultures of non-bronchoscopic samples in ventilator associated pneumonia. Indian J Med Microbiol,2006,24,107-13.
[9] Chastre, J. Conference summary: ventilator-associated pneumonia. Respir Care,2005,50,975-83.
[10] Meduri, GU; Mauldin, GL; Wunderink, RG; Leeper, KV, Jr.; Jones, CB; Tolley, E et al. Causes of fever and pulmonary densities in patients with clinical manifestations of ventilator-associated pneumonia. Chest,1994,106,221-35.
[11] Andrews, CP; Coalson, JJ; Smith, JD; Johanson, WG, Jr. Diagnosis of nosocomial bacterial pneumonia in acute, diffuse lung injury. Chest,1981,80,254-8.
[12] Fagon, JY; Chastre, J; Domart, Y; Trouillet, JL; Pierre, J; Darne C, et al. Nosocomial pneumonia in patients receiving continuous mechanical ventilation. Prospective analysis of 52 episodes with use of a protected specimen brush and quantitative culture techniques. Am Rev Respir Dis,1989,139,877-84.
[13] Meduri, GU; Wunderink, RG; Leeper, KV; Beals, DH. Management of bacterial pneumonia in ventilated patients. Protected bronchoalveolar lavage as a diagnostic tool. Chest,1992 ,101,500-8.
[14] Wunderink, RG; Woldenberg, LS; Zeiss, J; Day, CM; Ciemins, J; Lacher, DA. The radiologic diagnosis of autopsy-proven ventilator-associated pneumonia. Chest,1992,101,458-63.
[15] Chastre, J; Fagon, JY. Ventilator-associated pneumonia. Am J Respir Crit Care Med,2002 ,165,867-903.
[16] Koenig, SM; Truwit, JD. Ventilator-associated pneumonia: diagnosis, treatment, and prevention. Clin Microbiol Rev,2006, 19,637-57.
[17] Wunderink, RG. Radiologic diagnosis of ventilator-associated pneumonia. Chest,2000,117,188S-90S.
[18] Wunderink, RG. Clinical criteria in the diagnosis of ventilator-associated pneumonia. Chest,2000,117,191S-4S.
[19] Hunter, JD. Ventilator associated pneumonia. Postgrad Med J,2006,82,172-8.
[20] Alp, E; Voss, A. Ventilator associated pneumonia and infection control. Ann Clin Microbiol Antimicrob,2006,5:7.

[21] Fartoukh, M; Maitre, B; Honore, S; Cerf, C; Zahar, JR; Brun-Buisson, C. Diagnosing pneumonia during mechanical ventilation: the clinical pulmonary infection score revisited. Am J Respir Crit Care Med,2003,168,173-9.

[22] Niederman, MS. The clinical diagnosis of ventilator-associated pneumonia. Respir Care,2005 ,50,788-96.

[23] Johanson, WG, Jr.; Pierce, AK; Sanford, JP; Thomas, GD. Nosocomial respiratory infections with gram-negative bacilli. The significance of colonization of the respiratory tract. Ann Intern Med,1972,77,701-6.

[24] Fagon, JY; Chastre, J; Hance, AJ; Guiguet, M; Trouillet, JL; Domart, Y et al. Detection of nosocomial lung infection in ventilated patients. Use of a protected specimen brush and quantitative culture techniques in 147 patients. Am Rev Respir Dis,1988,138,110-6.

[25] Pugin, J; Auckenthaler, R; Mili, N; Janssens, JP; Lew, PD; Suter, PM. Diagnosis of ventilator-associated pneumonia by bacteriologic analysis of bronchoscopic and nonbronchoscopic "blind" bronchoalveolar lavage fluid. Am Rev Respir Dis,1991,143,1121-9.

[26] Torres, A; Carlet, J. Ventilator-associated pneumonia. European Task Force on ventilator-associated pneumonia. Eur Respir J,2001,17,1034-45.

[27] Gibot, S; Cravoisy, A; Levy, B; Bene, MC; Faure, G; Bollaert, PE. Soluble triggering receptor expressed on myeloid cells and the diagnosis of pneumonia. N Engl J Med,2004,350,451-8.

[28] Pelosi, P; Barassi, A; Severgnini, P; Gomiero, B; Finazzi, S; Merlini, G, et al. Prognostic role of clinical and laboratory criteria to identify early ventilator-associated pneumonia in brain injury. Chest,2008, 134,101-8.

[29] Timsit, JF; Cheval, C; Gachot, B; Bruneel, F; Wolff, M; Carlet, J et al. Usefulness of a strategy based on bronchoscopy with direct examination of bronchoalveolar lavage fluid in the initial antibiotic therapy of suspected ventilator-associated pneumonia. Intensive Care Med,2001,27,640-7.

[30] Singh, N; Rogers, P; Atwood, CW; Wagener, MM; Yu, VL. Short-course empiric antibiotic therapy for patients with pulmonary infiltrates in the intensive care unit. A proposed solution for indiscriminate antibiotic prescription. Am J Respir Crit Care Med,2000,162,505-11.

[31] Mayhall, CG. Ventilator-associated pneumonia or not? Contemporary diagnosis. Emerg Infect Dis,2001,7,200-4.

[32] Mertens, AH; Nagler, JM; Galdermans, DI; Slabbynck, HR; Weise, B; Coolen, D. Quality assessment of protected specimen brush samples by microscopic cell count. Am J Respir Crit Care Med,1998 ,157,1240-3.

[33] Blot, F; Raynard, B; Chachaty, E; Tancrede, C; Antoun, S; Nitenberg, G. Value of gram stain examination of lower respiratory tract secretions for early diagnosis of nosocomial pneumonia. Am J Respir Crit Care Med,2000,162,1731-7.

[34] Baughman, RP; Spencer, RE; Kleykamp, BO; Rashkin, MC; Douthit, MM. Ventilator associated pneumonia: quality of nonbronchoscopic bronchoalveolar lavage sample affects diagnostic yield. Eur Respir J,2000,16,1152-7.

[35] Baselski, VS; el-Torky, M; Coalson, JJ; Griffin, JP. The standardization of criteria for processing and interpreting laboratory specimens in patients with suspected ventilator-associated pneumonia. Chest,1992,102,571S-9S.

[36] Clec'h, C; Jaureguy, F; Hamza, L; Karoubi, P; Fosse, JP; Hamdi, A et al. Agreement between quantitative cultures of postintubation tracheal aspiration and plugged telescoping catheter, protected specimen brush, or BAL for the diagnosis of nosocomial pneumonia. Chest,2006,130,956-61.

[37] Wu, CL; Yang, DI; Wang, NY; Kuo, HT; Chen, PZ. Quantitative culture of endotracheal aspirates in the diagnosis of ventilator-associated pneumonia in patients with treatment failure. Chest,2002,122,662-8.

[38] Kahn, FW; Jones, JM. Diagnosing bacterial respiratory infection by bronchoalveolar lavage. J Infect Dis,1987,155,862-9.

[39] Salata, RA; Lederman, MM; Shlaes, DM; Jacobs, MR; Eckstein, E; Tweardy, D et al. Diagnosis of nosocomial pneumonia in intubated, intensive care unit patients. Am Rev Respir Dis,1987,135,426-32.

[40] Winn, WC; Allen, SD; Janda, WM; Koneman, EW; Procop, GW, Schreckenberger, PC et al. Koneman's Color Atlas and Textbook of Diagnostic Microbiology. 6th ed. Baltimore: Lippincott Williams & Wilkins; 2006.

[41] Brun-Buisson, C; Fartoukh, M; Lechapt, E; Honore, S; Zahar, JR; Cerf, C et al. Contribution of blinded, protected quantitative specimens to the diagnostic and therapeutic management of ventilator-associated pneumonia. Chest,2005,128,533-44.

[42] Morris, AJ; Tanner, DC; Reller, LB. Rejection criteria for endotracheal aspirates from adults. J Clin Microbiol,1993,31,1027-9.

[43] Kirtland, SH; Corley, DE; Winterbauer, RH; Springmeyer, SC; Casey, KR; Hampson, NB et al. The diagnosis of ventilator-associated pneumonia: a comparison of histologic, microbiologic, and clinical criteria. Chest,1997,112,445-57.

[44] Mertens, AH; Nagler, JM; Galdermans, DI; Slabbynck, HR; Weise, BS; Coolen, D. Diagnostic value of direct examination of protected specimen brush samples in nosocomial pneumonia. Eur J Clin Microbiol Infect Dis,1996 ,15,807-10.

[45] Duflo, F; Allaouchiche, B; Debon, R; Bordet, F; Chassard, D. An evaluation of the Gram stain in protected bronchoalveolar lavage fluid for the early diagnosis of ventilator-associated pneumonia. Anesth Analg,2001,92,442-7.

[46] Mimoz, O; Karim, A; Mazoit, JX; Edouard, A; Leprince, S; Nordmann, P. Gram staining of protected pulmonary specimens in the early diagnosis of ventilator-associated pneumonia. Br J Anaesth,2000,85,735-9.

[47] Sirvent, JM; Vidaur, L; Gonzalez, S; Castro, P; de, BJ; Castro, A et al. Microscopic examination of intracellular organisms in protected bronchoalveolar mini-lavage fluid for the diagnosis of ventilator-associated pneumonia. Chest,2003,123,518-23.

[48] Chastre, J; Fagon, JY; Bornet-Lecso, M;, Calvat, S; Dombret, MC; al, KR et al. Evaluation of bronchoscopic techniques for the diagnosis of nosocomial pneumonia. Am J Respir Crit Care Med,1995,152,231-40.

[49] Torres, A; El-Ebiary, M; Fabregas, N; Gonzalez, J; de la Bellacasa, JP; Hernandez, C et al. Value of intracellular bacteria detection in the diagnosis of ventilator associated pneumonia. Thorax,1996,51,378-84.

[50] Veber, B; Souweine, B; Gachot, B; Chevret, S; Bedos, JP; Decre, D et al. Comparison of direct examination of three types of bronchoscopy specimens used to diagnose nosocomial pneumonia. Crit Care Med,2000,28,962-8.

[51] Camargo, LF; De Marco, FV; Barbas, CS; Hoelz, C; Bueno, MA; Rodrigues, M, Jr. et al. Ventilator associated pneumonia: comparison between quantitative and qualitative cultures of tracheal aspirates. Crit Care,2004,R422-R430.

[52] Cook, D; Mandell L. Endotracheal aspiration in the diagnosis of ventilator-associated pneumonia. Chest,2000,117,195S-7S.

[53] Giantsou, E; Liratzopoulos, N; Efraimidou, E; Panopoulou, M; Alepopoulou, E; Kartali-Ktenidou, S et al. De-escalation therapy rates are significantly higher by bronchoalveolar lavage than by tracheal aspirate. Intensive Care Med,2007,33,1533-40.

[54] Baughman, RP. Diagnosis of ventilator-associated pneumonia. Microbes Infect,2005,7,262-7.

[55] The Canadian Critical Care Trials Group. A randomized trial of diagnostic techniques for ventilator-associated pneumonia. N Engl J Med,2006,355,2619-30.

[56] Aydogdu, M; Gursel, G; Hizel, K; Ozis, TN. Comparison of the serial surveillance with quantitative and non-quantitative tracheal aspirate in predicting ventilator-associated pneumonia etiology in patients receiving antibiotic therapy. Minerva Anestesiol,2010 ,76,600-8.

[57] Fujitani, S; Cohen-Melamed, MH; Tuttle, RP; Delgado, E; Taira, Y; Darby, JM. Comparison of semi-quantitative endotracheal aspirates to quantitative non-bronchoscopic bronchoalveolar lavage in diagnosing ventilator-associated pneumonia. Respir Care,2009,54,1453-61.

[58] Sauaia, A; Moore, FA; Moore, EE; Haenel, JB; Kaneer, L; Read, RA. Diagnosing pneumonia in mechanically ventilated trauma patients: endotracheal aspirate versus bronchoalveolar lavage. J Trauma,1993,35,512-7.

[59] Wood, AY; Davit, AJ; Ciraulo, DL; Arp, NW; Richart, CM; Maxwell, RA et al. A prospective assessment of diagnostic efficacy of blind protective bronchial brushings compared to bronchoscope-assisted lavage, bronchoscope-directed brushings, and blind endotracheal aspirates in ventilator-associated pneumonia. J Trauma,2003,55,825-34.

[60] Woske, HJ; Roding, T; Schulz, I; Lode, H. Ventilator-associated pneumonia in a surgical intensive care unit: epidemiology, etiology and comparison of three bronchoscopic methods for microbiological specimen sampling. Crit Care,2001,5,167-73.

[61] El Solh, AA; Akinnusi, ME; Pineda, LA; Mankowski, CR. Diagnostic yield of quantitative endotracheal aspirates in patients with severe nursing home-acquired pneumonia. Crit Care,2007,11,R57.

[62] Bergmans, DC; Bonten, MJ; de Leeuw, PW; Stobberingh, EE. Reproducibility of quantitative cultures of endotracheal aspirates from mechanically ventilated patients. J Clin Microbiol,1997,35,796-8.

[63] Sanchez-Nieto, JM; Torres, A; Garcia-Cordoba, F; El-Ebiary, M; Carrillo, A; Ruiz, J et al. Impact of invasive and noninvasive quantitative culture sampling on outcome of ventilator-associated pneumonia: a pilot study. Am J Respir Crit Care Med,1998,157,371-6.

[64] Luna, CM; Chirino, A. Qualitative cultures in ventilator-associated pneumonia - can they be used with confidence? Crit Care,2004,8,425-6.

[65] Sirvent, JM; Torres, A; Vidaur, L; Armengol, J; de, BJ; Bonet, A. Tracheal colonisation within 24 h of intubation in patients with head trauma: risk factor for developing early-onset ventilator-associated pneumonia. Intensive Care Med,2000,26,1369-72.

[66] Balthazar, AB; Von, NA; De Capitani, EM; Bottini, PV; Terzi, RG; Araujo, S. Diagnostic investigation of ventilator-associated pneumonia using bronchoalveolar lavage: comparative study with a postmortem lung biopsy. Braz J Med Biol Res,2001,34,993-1001.
[67] Meduri, GU; Chastre, J. The standardization of bronchoscopic techniques for ventilator-associated pneumonia. Chest,1992,102,557S-64S.
[68] Kollef, MH; Bock, KR; Richards, RD; Hearns, ML. The safety and diagnostic accuracy of minibronchoalveolar lavage in patients with suspected ventilator-associated pneumonia. Ann Intern Med,1995,122,743-8.
[69] Levy, H. Comparison of Ballard catheter bronchoalveolar lavage with bronchoscopic bronchoalveolar lavage. Chest,1994,106,1753-6.
[70] Joseph, NM; Sistla, S; Dutta, TK; Badhe, AS; Rasitha, D; Parija, SC. Role of semi-quantitative and quantitative cultures of endotracheal aspirates in the diagnosis of ventilator-associated pneumonia. Australasian Medical Journal,2010,In press.
[71] Grossman, RF; Fein, A. Evidence-based assessment of diagnostic tests for ventilator-associated pneumonia. Executive summary. Chest,2000,117,177S-81S.
[72] Gerbeaux, P; Ledoray, V; Boussuges, A; Molenat, F; Jean, P; Sainty, JM. Diagnosis of nosocomial pneumonia in mechanically ventilated patients: repeatability of the bronchoalveolar lavage. Am J Respir Crit Care Med,1998,157,76-80.
[73] Michel, F; Franceschini, B; Berger, P; Arnal, JM; Gainnier, M; Sainty, JM et al. Early antibiotic treatment for BAL-confirmed ventilator-associated pneumonia: a role for routine endotracheal aspirate cultures. Chest,2005,127,589-97.
[74] Delclaux, C; Roupie, E; Blot, F; Brochard, L; Lemaire, F; Brun-Buisson, C. Lower respiratory tract colonization and infection during severe acute respiratory distress syndrome: incidence and diagnosis. Am J Respir Crit Care Med,1997,156,1092-8.
[75] Joseph, NM; Sistla, S; Dutta, TK; Badhe, AS; Parija SC. Ventilator-associated pneumonia: role of colonizers and value of routine endotracheal aspirate cultures. Int J Infect Dis,2010,14,e723-e729.
[76] Hayon, J; Figliolini, C; Combes, A; Trouillet, JL; Kassis, N; Dombret, MC, et al. Role of serial routine microbiologic culture results in the initial management of ventilator-associated pneumonia. Am J Respir Crit Care Med,2002,165,41-6.
[77] Nopmaneejumruslers, C; Chan, CK. Is there a role for routine surveillance endotracheal aspirate cultures in the treatment of BAL-confirmed ventilator-associated pneumonia? Chest,2005,127,425-7.
[78] Katzenstein, AA; Askin, FB. Surgical pathology of non-neoplastic lung disease. 2nd ed. Philadelphia: W.B.Saunders; 1990.
[79] Rouby, JJ. Histology and microbiology of ventilator-associated pneumonias. Semin Respir Infect,1996,11,54-61.
[80] Torres, A; Fabregas, N; Ewig, S; de la Bellacasa, JP; Bauer, TT; Ramirez, J. Sampling methods for ventilator-associated pneumonia: validation using different histologic and microbiological references. Crit Care Med,2000,28,2799-804.
[81] Corley, DE; Kirtland, SH; Winterbauer, RH; Hammar, SP; Dail, DH, Bauermeister, DE et al. Reproducibility of the histologic diagnosis of pneumonia among a panel of four pathologists: analysis of a gold standard. Chest,1997,112,458-65.

[82] Marquette, CH; Wallet, F; Copin, MC; Wermert, D; Desmidt, A; Ramon, P et al. Relationship between microbiologic and histologic features in bacterial pneumonia. Am J Respir Crit Care Med,1996,154,1784-7.
[83] Chastre, J; Combes, A; Luyt,CE. The invasive (quantitative) diagnosis of ventilator-associated pneumonia. Respir Care,2005,50,797-807.
[84] Alfieri, N; Ramotar, K; Armstrong, P; Spornitz, ME; Ross, G; Winnick, J et al. Two consecutive outbreaks of Stenotrophomonas maltophilia (Xanthomonas maltophilia) in an intensive-care unit defined by restriction fragment-length polymorphism typing. Infect Control Hosp Epidemiol,1999,20,553-6.
[85] Joseph, NM; Sistla, S; Dutta, TK; Badhe, AS; Rasitha, D; Parija SC. Role of intensive care unit environment and health-care workers in transmission of ventilator-associated pneumonia. J Infect Dev Ctries,2010,4,282-91.
[86] Villers, D; Espaze, E; Coste-Burel, M; Giauffret, F; Ninin, E; Nicolas, F et al. Nosocomial Acinetobacter baumannii infections: microbiological and clinical epidemiology. Ann Intern Med,1998,129,182-9.
[87] Joseph, NM; Sistla, S; Dutta, TK; Badhe, AS; Parija, SC. Ventilator-associated pneumonia: A review. Eur J Intern Med,2010,doi:10.1016/j.ejim.2010.07.006.
[88] Luna, CM; Aruj, P; Niederman, MS; Garzon, J; Violi, D; Prignoni, A et al. Appropriateness and delay to initiate therapy in ventilator-associated pneumonia. Eur Respir J,2006,27,158-64.
[89] Joseph, NM; Sistla, S; Dutta, TK; Badhe, AS; Parija, SC. Outcome of ventilator-associated pneumonia: impact of appropriate therapy and other factors. Lung India,2010,In press.
[90] Rello, J; Paiva, JA; Baraibar, J; Barcenilla, F; Bodi, M; Castander, D et al. International Conference for the Development of Consensus on the Diagnosis and Treatment of Ventilator-associated Pneumonia. Chest,2001,120,955-70.
[91] Fowler, RA; Flavin, KE; Barr, J; Weinacker, AB; Parsonnet, J; Gould, MK. Variability in antibiotic prescribing patterns and outcomes in patients with clinically suspected ventilator-associated pneumonia. Chest,2003,123,835-44.
[92] Porzecanski, I; Bowton, DL. Diagnosis and treatment of ventilator-associated pneumonia. Chest,2006 ,130,597-604.
[93] Micek, ST; Ward, S; Fraser, VJ; Kollef, MH. A randomized controlled trial of an antibiotic discontinuation policy for clinically suspected ventilator-associated pneumonia. Chest,2004,125,1791-9.
[94] Afessa, B. From "pro and con" debate to evidence-based practice: ventilator-associated pneumonia. Chest,2004,125,1600-2.
[95] Kollef, MH; Kollef, KE. Antibiotic utilization and outcomes for patients with clinically suspected ventilator-associated pneumonia and negative quantitative BAL culture results. Chest,2005,128,2706-13.
[96] Dennesen, PJ; van d, V; Kessels, AG; Ramsay, G; Bonten, MJ. Resolution of infectious parameters after antimicrobial therapy in patients with ventilator-associated pneumonia. Am J Respir Crit Care Med, 2001,163,1371-5.
[97] Chastre, J; Wolff, M; Fagon, JY; Chevret, S; Thomas, F; Wermert, D et al. Comparison of 8 vs 15 days of antibiotic therapy for ventilator-associated pneumonia in adults: a randomized trial. JAMA,2003,290,2588-98.

[98] Kwa, AL; Loh, C; Low, JG; Kurup, A; Tam, VH. Nebulized colistin in the treatment of pneumonia due to multidrug-resistant Acinetobacter baumannii and Pseudomonas aeruginosa. Clin Infect Dis,2005,41,754-7.

[99] Brown, RB; Kruse, JA; Counts, GW; Russell, JA; Christou, NV; Sands, ML. Double-blind study of endotracheal tobramycin in the treatment of gram-negative bacterial pneumonia. The Endotracheal Tobramycin Study Group. Antimicrob Agents Chemother,1990,34,269-72.

[100] Hamer, DH. Treatment of nosocomial pneumonia and tracheobronchitis caused by multidrug-resistant Pseudomonas aeruginosa with aerosolized colistin. Am J Respir Crit Care Med,2000,162,328-30.

[101] MacIntyre, NR; Rubin, BK. Respiratory therapies in the critical care setting. Should aerosolized antibiotics be administered to prevent or treat ventilator-associated pneumonia in patients who do not have cystic fibrosis? Respir Care,2007,52,416-21.

[102] Klick, JM; du Moulin, GC; Hedley-Whyte, J; Teres, D; Bushnell, LS; Feingold, DS. Prevention of gram-negative bacillary pneumonia using polymyxin aerosol as prophylaxis. II. Effect on the incidence of pneumonia in seriously ill patients. J Clin Invest,1975,55,514-9.

In: Pneumonia: Symptoms, Diagnosis and Treatment
Editors: M. L. Suarez and S. M. Ortega, pp. 121-131
ISBN: 978-1-61209-685-8

Chapter V

Community Acquired Staphylococcal Pneumonia Complicating Influenza

Yoav Keynan and Ethan Rubinstein*
University of Manitoba, Winnipeg, Canada

Abstract

Bacterial pneumonia complicating influenza has been recognized at least since the 19th century. In this setting Staphylococcus aureus is one of the most common offenders and is associated with a potentially severe disease accompanied by high rates of morbidity and mortality. The recent increase in staphylococcal infections caused by community-acquired methicillin-resistant Staphylococcus aureus (CA-MRSA), has been increasingly recognized to be associated with community associated pneumonia (CAP) This type of pneumonia affects mainly a younger age group, frequently follows infection with influenza, and is often severe, requiring hospitalization and causing death in a significant proportion of those affected. Recognizing the role of Staphylococcus aureus in general and CA-MRSA in particular as important causes of pneumonia after influenza infection may decrease the delay before the institution of appropriate antimicrobial therapy, which in turn should contribute to improved outcome of this severe disease. This article reviews the epidemiology, clinical features, diagnosis, and therapies for staphylococcal pneumonia complicating influenza virus infection. Staphylococcus aureus (SA) is a relatively uncommon cause of community acquired pneumonia thought to account for only 3–5% of cases [1, 2]. S. aureus pneumonia is, however, a well-recognized complication occurring after infection with influenza both following seasonal and pandemic types and other viral pneumonia (varicella, adeno-virus) in children and young adults. S. aureus pneumonia complicating influenza has accounted for a large number of deaths [3–6]. Morens et al. reviewed bacterial culture results from 96 autopsy series, from civil and military sources from the 1918-1919 influenza pandemic, a total of 5266 positive culture results- were found. S. aureus was the third most common bacterial

* Correspondence: Ethan Rubinstein, MD, LLB, Section of Infectious Diseases, Faculty of Medicine, University of Manitoba, 543-730 William Avenue, 501 Basic Medical Sciences Building, Winnipeg, MB R3E 0W3, Canada. Phone: 1-204-977-5680-1 Fax: 1-204-789-3926 E-mail: erubins@yahoo.com

pathogen identified, accounting for 8.1% of deaths occurring in these series [7]. Recent data is emerging to suggest an increase in the frequency of SA pneumonia. Possibly the first documented cases in North America were reported by Francis et. al[8]. All 4 patients in that small case series had a syndrome characterized by an influenza or influenza-like prodrome, shock and cavitary lesion. One of the patients succumbed to the infections while the others recovered after a prolonged hospital course Finelli et al.[9] reported 166 influenza- associated pediatric deaths in the years 2004-2007 pointing to the seriousness of this super-infection. Reports of bacterial co-infection of influenza increased from 6% in 2004–2005, to 15% in 2005-2006 and to 34% in 2006–2007. S aureus was isolated from a sterile site or from the endotracheal tube in 1 case in 2004–2005, from 3 cases in 2005–2006, and from 22 cases in 2006–2007. Another trend observed in this study was the significant role of methicillin-resistant S aureus (MRSA) accounting for 64% of SA isolates, with the majority of cases occurring in the latest reporting period [9]. A survey of 59 US hospitals involving 4543 patients with culture-positive pneumonia between January 2002 and January 2004 [10] identified MRSA as a potential pathogen in CAP (8.9%). Moreover, Staphylococcus aureus was the only pathogen identified to be independently associated with mortality according to a logistic regression analysis in this study. Kallen et al. [11] reported a survey conducted by The Infectious Diseases Society of America's Emerging Infections Network (EIN) in 2007, revealing episodes of severe S. aureus community acquired pneumonia (CAP) diagnosed during the 2006-2007 influenza season. CAP was defined as "pneumonia requiring hospitalization of an outpatient not residing in a long-term care facility." Nearly half of the responding surveyed members (509- 47%) reported treating a total of 440 adults and 117 children who were hospitalized because of S. aureus CAP. Of these patients, nearly a half (49%) required mechanical ventilation, and 13% succumbed to the infection. In the survey, respondents suspected that a quarter of the patients had an associated influenza infection, on basis of history or clinical findings. However, influenza was confirmed by laboratory testing in only 6% of cases. This report too points to the increased frequency and severity of S A pneumonia complicating viral pneumonia.

The CDC has documented reports from state and local health departments over the last several

influenza seasons describing previously healthy children with a severe s. aureus CAP [12]. The increasing role of CA-MRSA and high mortality rates are evident in more recent reports, although it is unclear whether they represent heightened awareness and reporting or a real shift in severity.

The mechanisms by which prior influenza infection predisposes to subsequent SA pneumonia is beyond the scope of this manuscript and may involve changes in epithelial defense and changes in epithelial cell wall leading to increased bacterial adherence, changes in the ability of the innate cells to recognize the pathogen, impaired migration or inability of macrophages and white blood cells to eradicate the invading organism [13-15]. The magnitude of the risk depends on the particular strain of influenza virus and the degree of local epithelial damage and immune dysregulation the viral infection induces as well as on the virulence and antibiotic susceptibility of the ensuing SA strains.

Clinical Features

Identifying the unique features of SA pneumonia occurring after influenza virus infection is hampered by the usual lack of a laboratory proof for the identity of the viral infection at the time of presentation to the health care system. Pneumonia in young, previously healthy adults with a preceding influenza-like illness characterized by severe respiratory symptoms, hemoptysis, high fever, leukopenia, very high C-reactive protein (>400 G/L), hypotension, and a chest x-ray showing multilobular cavitating alveolar infiltrates should lead one to suspect CA-MRSA infection [16-22] (Figure 1). Some cases are further complicated by empyema and pneumothorax or pyo-pneumothorax and may culminate in ARDS. Young age has been a consistent feature of CA-MRSA pneumonia in both the European and US series [16,17,23]. Importantly, preceding influenza or influenza-like illness has been described in 75% of cases. [16,17]. The severity of these pneumonias is demonstrated by the fact that in one series, 81% of hospitalized patients needed admission to the intensive care unit, 62% required intubation, 46% had chest tube placement, and 29% died [17].

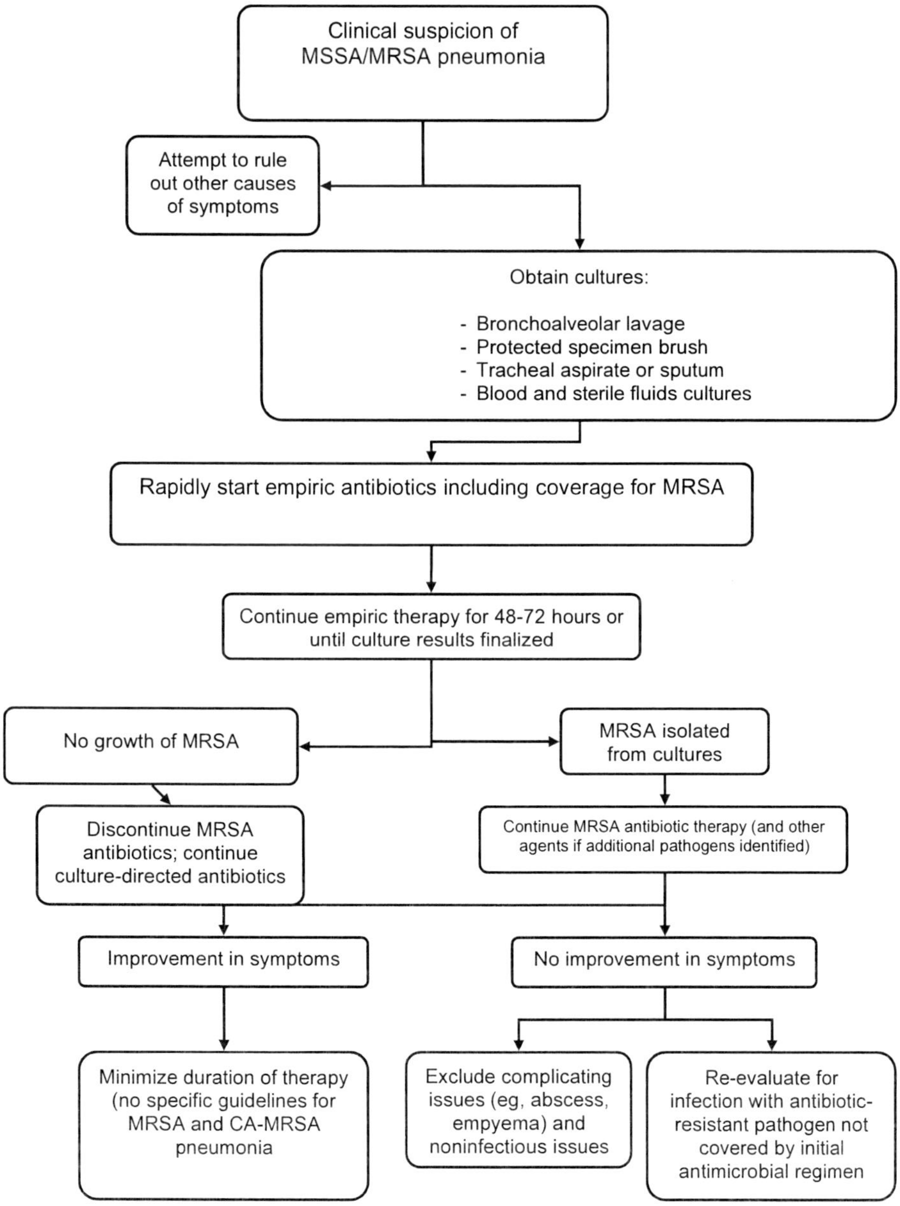

Figure 1. Management of patient with suspected staphylococcal pneumonia.

The CDC reported a series of 10 additional cases of MRSA CAP from the southern United States affecting young, healthy, patients with preceding influenza or influenza-like illnesses [12]. Six of the 10 patients died after a mean of only 3.5 days from the onset of symptoms. All tested MRSA isolates (5/10) were positive for the Panton Valentine Leucocidin (=PVL) and carried the SCCmec type IVa cassette. All isolates had indistinguishable pulse field electrophoresis pattern, belonged to the USA 300-0114 clone, and were resistant to beta-lactams and erythromycin; 2 strains had inducible resistance to clindamycin, and 2 were levofloxacin non-susceptible [12]. Gillet et al. examined the factors predicting mortality in a prospective study of 50 cases with necrotizing pneumonia caused by PVL producing SA, identified by the French National Reference for Staphylococci. They found that deaths, as previously shown were associated with septic shock and respiratory failure and were predicted by airway bleeding, erythroderma and leukopenia [24].

Diagnosis

The clinical diagnosis of community-acquired staphylococcal pneumonia is frequently difficult. In some cases of staphylococcal pneumonia, a history of preceding upper respiratory or influenza-like illness could be elicited, however influenza is relatively infrequently documented. Conversely, documentation of staphylococcal pneumonia in individuals admitted for severe influenza is more frequent but often represents a complication of hospital admission and respiratory support, that is, a nosocomial infection of the hospital Acquired Pneumonia type (HAP) or Ventilatory Associated Pneumonia (VAP) type. Strangely, and even after the recent H1N1 outbreak and the occasional presence of H5N1 cases the current Infectious Diseases Society of America/American Thoracic Society, Canadian and British Thoracic Society guidelines do not include preceding influenza infection in the list of indications for extensive diagnostic testing [25,26,27]. An update of these guidelines would likely address these issues. Presently therefore, a high level of suspicion is probably the most important factor in establishing an early rapid diagnosis.

CA-MRSA should be suspected as the cause of CAP in the presence of the following key features: influenza-like prodrome, hemoptysis [24], severe respiratory symptoms, high fever, leukopenia, hypotension, and a chest x-ray showing multilobular infiltrates, with or without cavitation in addition to an appropriate epidemiological background particularly in a patient with aprecceding skin or soft tissue infection known to be caused by MRSA [11].

Therapy

The first, and arguably the most important, aspect of treatment is the need for rapid institution of appropriate antibiotic therapy. This principle has been demonstrated by Kumar et al [28] demonstrating that in septic and hypotensive patients, each hour delay in therapy was associated with an increase in mortality of 6.3%. Similarly, Kim et al demonstrated that delay of effective therapy in patients with MRSA bacteremia and noneradicable foci of infection, which includes pneumonia, was associated with increased mortality [29]. The current guidelines for treatment of community acquired pneumonia do not typically provide adequate coverage for MRSA, hence delay with potential deleterious consequences may ensue.

Pneumonia Caused by Methicillin-susceptible Staphylococcus aureus

Pneumonia caused by MSSA strains containing MRSA has been described as clinically indistinguishable from CA MRSA pneumonia containing PVL, both organisms affecting young individuals and are associated with multi-lobe presentation, leucopenia, severe prostration, very high mortality and an exceedingly rapid course (30). While previous reports suggested that MSSA pneumonia should never be treated with vancomycin as the mortality of this disease is very high with this treatment (50%) and that beta-lactam antibiotics are the preferable agents in MSSA pneumonia (31, 32), in recent years there is some change in this position. That is, vancomycin is still not indicated for such MSSA patients but new data suggest that such patients may benefit from combination therapy of beta-lactam antibiotic in combination with linezolid or clindamycin or rifampin, or conversely be treated with linezolid or clindamycin alone (33,34, 35,36). The reason being that cloxacillin and other beta lactam antibiotics that bind to the Penicillin Bounding Protein 1, (=PBP-1) increase the production of PVL, while beta lactam antibiotics that bind to PBP 2-4 do not alter PVL production (37). Furthermore, linezolid, clindamycin and rifampin reduce the in vitro production of PVL compared to non treated S.aureus cells and even the enhanced production of PVL induced by cloxacillin whereas aminoglycosides, vancomycin, quinupristin/dalfopristin are neutral vis a vis PVL production (37, 38,39). Other investigators believe that PVL has no decisive role in the pathogenesis and other staphylococcal toxigenic factors like superantigens, α- toxin, hemolysins, enterotoxins, phenol soluble protein (PSM), δ-toxin, and the Agr system (the operon that regulates gene expression) are more important or equally important to the PVL in causing the extensive damage to the lungs seen in such cases (40,41, 42).

Presently acceptable treatment should include a beta-lactam antibiotic and in suspected PVL carrying S.aureus of the MSSA type responsible for the infection that addition of linezolid or clindamycin should be considered as first line therapy. In beta-lactam allergic individuals, consideration should be given to the use of linezolid as a single agent, or, in the future telavancin.

Pneumonia Caused by Methicillin-resistant Staphylococcus aureus

MRSA pneumonia needs to be divided into Community originating CAP caused by CA MRSA, particularly the strain USA 300 and nosocomial pneumonia causing HAP and VAP.

CA MRSA causing CAP can be a highly lethal disease as described previously (16,17). The organisms causing the disease are equipped with a variety of enzymes and toxins to cause a rapid irreversible damage of the alveolar epithelial cells. It is therefore advisable to use in such instances antibiotics that in addition to their antimicrobial properties might antagonize or diminish toxin production or secretion from the bacterial cells. Classically, clindamycin has been recommended for such purposes both in streptococcal and staphylococcal infections and was recently shown to inhibit PVL production (37-39). Anecdotal cases also document the reversal of seemingly very severe pneumonia when such an agent was used (33). Clindamycin does not uniquely possess this activity, but also rifampin and linezolid have been shown to have such anti-PVL properties, this may account for additional isolated case reports favouring the use of these agents or vancomycin and other glycopeptides in CA MRSA causing CAP, particularly in younger individuals and un children who are desperately sick (36,43, 44 ,45). An additional available therapeutic option is to use IVIG which contains antibodies against staphylococcal toxin and enzymes and particularly against the superantigen, however experience is still lacking concerning the effects of such 'old' therapeutic modality.

In HAP and VAP the situation seems to be different, hospital originating MRSA usually do not possess the machinery that community MRSA have to attack the host so violently. HAP and VAP are often caused by MRSA in conjunction with Gram-negative pathogens, frequently with reduced antimicrobial susceptibility to conventional antibiotics. Thus the clinical outcome relies on an appropriate combination of effective anti MRSA agents in combination with effective Gram-negative coverage. Numerous clinical trials comparing various antibiotics active against MRSA failed to show statistically significant superiority of any agent over vancomycin in both HAP and VAP. Agents studied recently include: ceftobiprole, oritavancin, telavancin tigecycline iclaprim and linezolid (45, 46, 47 ,48, 49, 50) . Several trials however demonstrated numerical superiority over vancomycin in various subsets of patients. On the other hand in view of the recently reported 'vancomycin creep' particularly in the US but also globally (51, 52, 53) and the reduced therapeutic effects in infections caused by MRSA with elevated vancomycin MIC > 1.0 mg/L (54, 55) it seems reasonable to use an alternative therapy in geographical areas which experience the 'vancomycin creep'. Options would include telavancin which showed superiority over vancomycin in subset of patients with elevated vancomycin MIC's (47) or linezolid or tigecycline. There is no place for combination therapy against MRSA in HAP and VAP as the results of single agents are satisfactory. Of note is that daptomycin, despite its excellent in vitro activity and rapid killing should under no circumstances be used in HAP and VAP caused by MRSA due to its inactivation by surfactant (56). Recent development in this field is the use of intra-tracheally administered antibiotics for the control of resistant infections. This new application route allows for the delivery of very high drug concentrations deep into the lung with the hope to overcome resistance, to deliver high drug concentrations into infected areas overcoming the antagonistic impact of pus, low pH, white cell break products etc' which impair the antibacterial activity of many antibiotics that reach the lungs following systemic administration. Early experiences with intrattracheal amikacin, intratracheal aztreonam ,intratracheal polymyxin and intratracheal fluoroquinolones are encouraging although most are aimed at Gram-negative pathogens.

Duration and Modification of Therapy

Because unnecessarily broad-spectrum antibiotic therapy promotes the emergence of resistant organisms in individual patients and the environment, modification of the initial broad-spectrum antibiotic regimen administered empirically to patients with HCAP, HAP, and VAP using a de-escalation strategy should occur when possible. De-escalation should be based on the patient's clinical response as well as on microbiologic results (especially quantitative lower respiratory cultures) and change in the clinical pulmonary infection score

(CPIS). Modification should include decreasing the number and/or spectrum of antibiotics, shortening the duration of therapy in patients who have uncomplicated infections and are demonstrating signs of clinical improvement, and discontinuing antibiotics altogether in patients who have a noninfectious etiology identified for their clinical event. Kollef and colleagues [50] found that patients with a clinical suspicion for VAP and culture-negative BAL results for a major pathogen or a CPIS of ≤ 6 on day 3 could have their antimicrobial therapy safely discontinued [51,52]. Similarly, several clinical trials have found that 7 to 8 days of antibiotic treatment is acceptable for most non-bacteremic patients with VAP [53]. However, the duration of therapy for MRSA-caused HAP or VAP needs additional evaluation since the studies that evaluated treatment duration included insufficient numbers of MRSA-infected patients [53,54]. As a result, presently the duration of therapy for nonbacteremic MRSA should be based on clinical judgment; most investigators would provide a minimum of 10-14 days of therapy. For patients with bacteremic MRSA pneumonia, duration of therapy must take into consideration the potential for complicated bacteremia with metastatic foci of infection (endocarditis and osteomyelitis), necessitaiting a more prolonged course of antibiotic therapy. Based on the available evidence, the suggested management of a patient with suspected staphylococcal pneumonia is depicted in Figure 1.

Conclusions

Staphylococcus aureus is an uncommon cause of community–acquired pneumonia, however it is one of the leading causes of pneumonia occurring after influenza virus infection. Recent reports document an increase in the frequency of SA pneumonia and the spread of CA-MRSA has been accompanied by a rise in the incidence of severe pneumonia attributed to this pathogen. The current guidelines do not reflect the significant role that SA has in CAP complicating influenza and the limited recommended diagnostic tests for CAP will frequently fail to identify this organism. The ensuing antimicrobial therapy recommended by the same guidelines frequently does not provide coverage for this etiologic agent. It is therefore high index of suspicion that is relied upon for making the diagnosis of SA and for institution of antimicrobial therapy that provides coverage for CA-MRSA.

References

[1] Ruiz M, et al. Etiology of community-acquired pneumonia: impact of age, comorbidity, and severity. American Journal of Respiratory and Critical Care Medicine 1999; 160: 397–405.

[2] Stankovic C, Mahajan P, Asmar BI. Methicillin resistant Staphylococcus aureus as a cause of community- acquired pneumonia. Current Infectious Disease Reports 2007; 9: 223–227.

[3] Chickering HT, Park JH. Staphylococcus aureus pneumonia. New England Journal of Medicine 1919; 72:617–626.

[4] Robertson L, Caley JP, Moore J. Importance of Staphylococcus aureus in pneumonia in the 1957 epidemic of influenza A. Lancet 1958; 2: 233–236.

[5] Martin CM, et al. Asian influenza A in Boston, 1957–58. Archives of Internal Medicine 1959; 103: 532–542.

[6] Bhat N, et al. Influenza-associated deaths among children in the United States, 2003–2004. New England Journal of Medicine 2005; 353: 2559–2567.

[7] Morens DM, Taubenburger JK, Fauci AS (2008) Predominant role of bacterial pneumonia as a cause of death in pandemic influenza: implications for pandemic influenza preparedness. J Infect Dis 198: 962–70.

[8] Francis, J. S., M. C. Doherty, U. Lopatin, C. P. Johnston, G. Sinha, T. Ross, M. Cai, et al. 2005. Severe community-onset pneumonia in healthy adults caused by methicillin-resistant staphylococcus aureus carrying the panton-valentine leukocidin genes. Clinical Infectious Diseases 2005;40 (1): 100-7.

[9] Finelli L, et al. Influenza-associated pediatric mortality in the United States : increase of Staphylococcus aureus coinfection. Pediatrics 2008; 122: 805–811.

[10] Kollef MH, Shorr A, Tabak YP, Gupta V, Liu LZ, Johannes RS. Epidemiology and outcomes of health-care-associated pneumonia: results from a large US database of culture-positive pneumonia. Chest 2005; 128:3854-62.

[11] Kallen AJ, et al. Characteristics of Staphylococcus aureus community-acquired pneumonia during the 2006–2007 influenza season. Clinical Infectious Diseases 2007; 45: 1655.

[12] Centers for Disease Control and Prevention. Severe methicillin-resistant Staphylococcus aureus community acquired pneumonia associated with influenza – Louisiana and Georgia, December 2006–January2007. Morbidity and Mortality Weekly Report 2008; 25: 325–329.

[13] Didierlaurent, A., J. Goulding, and T. Hussell. 2007. The impact of successive infections on the lung microenvironment. *Immunology* 122 (4) (Dec): 457-65.

[14] Mao, H., W. Tu, Y. Liu, G. Qin, J. Zheng, P. L. Chan, K. T. Lam, J. S. Peiris, and Y. L. Lau. 2010. Inhibition of human natural killer cell activity by influenza virions and hemagglutinin. *Journal of Virology* 84 (9) (May): 4148-57.

[15] Meunier, I., S. Pillet, J. N. Simonsen, and V. von Messling. 2010. Influenza pathogenesis: Lessons learned from animal studies with H5N1, H1N1 spanish, and pandemic H1N1 2009 influenza. *Critical Care Medicine* 38 (4 Suppl) (Apr): e21-9.

[16] Gillet Y, Issartel B, Vanhems P, et al. Association between *Staphylococcus aureus* strains carrying gene for Panton-Valentine leukocidin and highly lethal necrotising pneumonia in young immunocompetent patients. Lancet 2002; 359:753-9.

[17] Hageman JC, Uyeki TM, Francis JS, et al. Severe community-acquired pneumonia due to *Staphylococcus aureus*, 2003-04 influenza season. Emerg Infect Dis 2006; 12:894-9.

[18] Morgan M. *Staphylococcus aureus*, Panton-Valentine leukocidin, and necrotising pneumonia. BMJ 2005; 331:793-4.

[19] Wargo KA, Eiland EH, III. Appropriate antimicrobial therapy for community-acquired methicillin-resistant *Staphylococcus aureus* carrying the Panton-Valentine leukocidin genes. Clin Infect Dis 2005; 40:1376-8.

[20]Monaco M, Antonucci R, Palange P, Venditti M, Pantosti A. Methicillin-resistant *Staphylococcus aureus* necrotizing pneumonia. Emerg Infect Dis 2005; 11:1647-8.

[21]Peleg AY, Munckhof WJ. Fatal necrotising pneumonia due to community-acquired methicillin-resistant *Staphylococcus aureus* (MRSA). Med J Aust 2004; 181:228-9.

[22] Micek ST, Dunne M, Kollef MH. Pleuropulmonary complications of Panton-Valentine leukocidin-positive community-acquired methicillin-resistant *Staphylococcus aureus*: Importance of treatment with antimicrobials inhibiting exotoxin production. Chest 2005; 128:2732-8.
[23] Gonzalez BE, Hulten KG, Dishop MK, et al. Pulmonary manifestations in children with invasive community-acquired *Staphylococcus aureus* infection. Clin Infect Dis 2005; 41:583-90.
[24] Gillet Y, Vanhems P, Lina G, Bes M, Vandenesch F, Floret D, Etienne J. Factors predicting mortality in necrotizing community-acquired pneumonia caused by Staphylococcus aureus containing Panton-Valentine leukocidin. Clin Infect Dis. 2007 Aug 1;45(3):315-21.
[25] Lim, W. S., S. V. Baudouin, R. C. George, A. T. Hill, C. Jamieson, I. Le Jeune, J. T. Macfarlane, et al. 2009. BTS guidelines for the management of community acquired pneumonia in adults: Update 2009. Thorax 64 Suppl 3 (Oct): iii1-55.
[26] Mandell, L. A., T. J. Marrie, R. F. Grossman, A. W. Chow, R. H. Hyland, and The Canadian CAP Working Group. 2000. Summary of canadian guidelines for the initial management of community-acquired pneumonia: An evidence-based update by the canadian infectious disease society and the canadian thoracic society. The Canadian Journal of Infectious Diseases = Journal Canadien Des Maladies Infectieuses 11 (5) (Sep): 237-48.
[27] Mandell, L. A., R. G. Wunderink, A. Anzueto, J. G. Bartlett, G. D. Campbell, N. C. Dean, S. F. Dowell, et al. 2007. Infectious diseases society of America/American thoracic society consensus guidelines on the management of community-acquired pneumonia in adults. Clin Infect Dis 2007: 44 Suppl 2 (Mar 1): S27-72.
[28] Kumar A, Roberts D, Wood KE, et al. Duration of hypotension before initiation of effective antimicrobial therapy is the critical determinant of survival in human septic shock. Crit Care Med 2006; 34:1589-96.
[29] Kim SH, Park WB, Lee KD, et al. Outcome of *Staphylococcus aureus* bacteremia in patients with eradicable foci versus noneradicable foci. Clin Infect Dis 2003; 37:794-9.
[30] Vardakas KZ, Matthaiou DK, Falagas ME Comparison of community-acquired pneumonia due to methicillin-resistant and methicillin-susceptible Staphylococcus aureus producing the Panton-Valentine leukocidin. Int J Tuberc Lung Dis. 2009 ;13:1476-85.
[31] González C, Rubio M, Romero-Vivas J, González M, Picazo JJ Bacteremic pneumonia due to Staphylococcus aureus: A comparison of disease caused by methicillin-resistant and methicillin-susceptible organisms Clin Infect Dis. 1999 ;5:1171-7.
[32] Rello J, Torres A, Ricart M, Valles J, Gonzalez J, Artigas A, Rodriguez-Roisin R. Ventilator-associated pneumonia by Staphylococcus aureus. Comparison of methicillin-resistant and methicillin-sensitive episodes. Am J Respir Crit Care Med. 1994 150(6 Pt 1):1545-9
[33] Rouzic N, Janvier F, Libert N, Javouhey E, Lina G, Nizou JY, Pasquier P, Stamm D, Brinquin L, Pelletier C, Vandenesch F, Floret D, Etienne J, Gillet Y. Prompt and successful toxin-targeting treatment of three patients with necrotizing pneumonia due to Staphylococcus aureus strains carrying the Panton-Valentine leukocidin genes. J Clin Microbiol. 2010;48;:1952-5.

[34] Pasquier P, Muller V, Villevieille T, Rousseau JM, Janvier F, Etienne J. Panton-Valentine leukocidin-producing Staphylococcus aureus necrotising pneumonia: measuring toxin levels in microbiological samples to attest of linezolid clinical efficacy. Int J Antimicrob Agents. 2010 ;35:613-4

[35] Kollef MH, Rello J, Cammarata SK, Croos-Dabrera RV, Wunderink RG. Clinical cure and survival in Gram-positive ventilator-associated pneumonia: retrospective analysis of two double-blind studies comparing linezolid with vancomycin. Intensive Care Med. 2004 ;30:388-94

[36] Hidron AI, Low CE, Honig EG, Blumberg HM Emergence of community-acquired meticillin-resistant Staphylococcus aureus strain USA300 as a cause of necrotising community-onset pneumonia. Lancet Infect Dis. 2009 ;9:384-92

[37] Dumitrescu O, Badiou C, Bes M, Reverdy ME, Vandenesch F, Etienne J, Lina G. Effect of antibiotics, alone and in combination, on Panton-Valentine leukocidin production by a Staphylococcus aureus reference strain. Clin Microbiol Infect. 2008 ;14:384-8

[38] Dumitrescu O, Boisset S, Badiou C, Bes M, Benito Y, Reverdy ME, Vandenesch F, Etienne J, Lina G. Effect of antibiotics on Staphylococcus aureus producing Panton-Valentine leukocidin. Antimicrob Agents Chemother. 2007 ;51:1515-9

[39] Dumitrescu O, Badiou C, Bes M, Reverdy ME, Vandenesch F, Etienne J, Lina G. Effect of antibiotics, alone and in combination, on Panton-Valentine leukocidin production by a Staphylococcus aureus reference strain. Clin Microbiol Infect. 2008 ;14:384-8.

[40] Schlievert PM. Cytolysins, superantigens, and pneumonia due to community-associated methicillin-resistant Staphylococcus aureus. J Infect Dis. 2009 ;200:676-8.

[41] Huseby M, Shi K, Brown CK, Digre J, Mengistu F, Seo KS, Bohach GA, Schlievert PM, Ohlendorf DH, Earhart CA. Structure and biological activities of beta toxin from Staphylococcus aureus. J Bacteriol. 2007;189:8719-26

[42] Otto M. Novel targeted immunotherapy approaches for staphylococcal infection. Expert Opin Biol Ther. 2010 ;10:1049-59.

[43] Lobo LJ, Reed KD, Wunderink RG Expanded clinical presentation of community-acquired methicillin-resistant Staphylococcus aureus pneumonia. Chest. 2010 ;138:130-6

[44] Marcinak JF, Frank AL. Treatment of community-acquired methicillin-resistant Staphylococcus aureus in children. Curr Opin Infect Dis. 2003 ;16:265-9.

[45] Dauner DG, Nelson RE, Taketa DC Ceftobiprole: A novel, broad-spectrum cephalosporin with activity against methicillin-resistant Staphylococcus aureus Am J Health Syst Pharm. 2010;67 45:983-93.

[46] Neuner EA, Ritchie DJ, Micek ST. New antibiotics for healthcare-associated pneumonia. Semin Respir Crit Care Med. 2009 ;30:92-101

[47] Rubinstein E, Lalani T, Corey GR, Kanafani ZA, Nannini EC, Rocha MG, Rahav G, Niederman MS, Kollef MH, Shorr AF, Lee P,. Lentnek AL, Luna CM, Jean-Yves Fagon, Torres A, Kitt MM, Genter FC, Barriere SL, Friedland HD,. Stryjewski ME, for the ATTAIN Study Group. Telavancin versus Vancomycin for Hospital-Acquired Pneumonia due to Gram-positive Pathogens Accepted for publication Clinical Infectious Diseases

[48] Freire AT, Melnyk V, Kim MJ, Datsenko O, Dzyublik O, Glumcher F, Chuang YC, Maroko RT, Dukart G, Cooper CA, Korth-Bradley JM, Dartois N, Gandjini H; for the 311 Study Group. Comparison of tigecycline with imipenem/cilastatin for the treatment of hospital-acquired pneumonia. Diagn Microbiol Infect Dis. 2010 ;68:140-151

[49] Rubinstein E, Cammarata S, Oliphant T, Wunderink R; Linezolid Nosocomial Pneumonia Study Group Linezolid (PNU-100766) versus vancomycin in the treatment of hospitalized patients with nosocomial pneumonia: a randomized, double-blind, multicenter study. Clin Infect Dis. 2001 ;32:402-12.

[50] Wunderink RG, Rello J, Cammarata SK, Croos-Dabrera RV, Kollef MH Linezolid vs vancomycin: analysis of two double-blind studies of patients with methicillin-resistant Staphylococcus aureus nosocomial pneumonia. Chest. 2003;124:1789-97

[51] Steinkraus G, White R, Friedrich L. Vancomycin MIC creep in non-vancomycin-intermediate Staphylococcus aureus (VISA), vancomycin-susceptible clinical methicillin-resistant S. aureus (MRSA) blood isolates from 2001-05. J Antimicrob Chemother. 2007;60:788-94.

[52] Ho PL, Lo PY, Chow KH, Lau EH, Lai EL, Cheng VC, Kao RY.Vancomycin MIC creep in MRSA isolates from 1997 to 2008 in a healthcare region in Hong Kong. J Infect. 2010;60:140-5

[53] Sakoulas G, Moellering RC Jr Increasing antibiotic resistance among methicillin-resistant Staphylococcus aureus strains. Clin Infect Dis. 2008 Suppl 5:S360-7.

[54] Soriano A, Marco F, Martínez JA, Pisos E, Almela M, Dimova VP, Alamo D, Ortega M, Lopez J, Mensa J. Influence of vancomycin minimum inhibitory concentration on the treatment of methicillin-resistant Staphylococcus aureus bacteremia. Clin Infect Dis. 2008 ;46:193-200

[55] Sakoulas G, Moise-Broder PA, Schentag J, Forrest A, Moellering RC Jr, Eliopoulos GM. Relationship of MIC and bactericidal activity to efficacy of vancomycin for treatment of methicillin-resistant Staphylococcus aureus bacteremia. J Clin Microbiol. 2004 ;42:2398-402

[56] Silverman JA, Mortin LI, Vanpraagh AD, Li T, Alder J. Inhibition of daptomycin by pulmonary surfactant: in vitro modeling and clinical impact. J Infect Dis. 2005 191:2149-52.

In: Pneumonia: Symptoms, Diagnosis and Treatment
Editors: M. L. Suarez and S. M. Ortega, pp. 133-149
ISBN: 978-1-61209-685-8

Chapter VI

Radiological Manifestations of Pneumonia in Common Practice: An Etiological Approach according to the Host

Angel Daniel Dominguez-Perez, Victoria Carnerero-Herrera, Cristina Martinez-Polanco, Raquel Gonzalez-Martin and Mª Alcazar Iribarren-Marin
Radiology Department, Virgen del Rocio University Hospital, Seville, Spain

Pulmonary infections still remain the most common infectious cause of mortality in the world, causing around six million deaths per year in the United States where they are the sixth cause of mortality and an important morbid-mortality source. We are therefore facing a problem enormous magnitude in social, economic and above all, health service areas.

In this chapter we will refer to pneumonia as an inflammatory-infectious process, although it is necessary to be aware of the existence of other etiological causes of inflammation in the lung that are not specifically mentioned in this chapter. When we find a patient presenting fever, cough, tachypnea, and rales on auscultation a clinical diagnosis of infectious pneumonia should be considered although at the same time we know that there are certain pathologies that can clinically mimic the presence of pneumonia. To guide the clinical diagnosis of pneumonia, establish the optimal treatment based on the etiological diagnosis and make an adequate follow up of these patients various diagnostic tests, both invasive and non-invasive, are available to us. Among the complete diagnostic battery used to the study lung infections the 'Gold Standard' test is currently the conventional chest radiograph (CXR). In fact, the American Thoracic Society recommends the practice of a CXR, including posterior/anterior and lateral projectionsfor an adult with suspected pneumonia [(1)]. So this is the first step that we must take. Just a single study composed of two projections of the patient's chest that will give us valuable information for an initial interpretation. If there is no clinical-radiological correlation or we find complications or abnormal evolution of the infection we can carry out Computed Tomography (CT) or other useful procedures for the management of the pneumonia. Within the range of available non-invasive laboratory tests we should mention sputum and blood culture or serology of infectious agents. On the invasive side we can use transtracheal aspiration, thoracentesis, closed pleural biopsy, bronchoscopy with aspiration and brushing, transbronchial biopsy, percutaneous aspiration and open pulmonary or pleural biopsies.

Sometimes pneumonia can be a difficult radiological diagnosis, either because of unclear initial findings or its masking by inflammatory complications such as pleural effusion, pulmonary edema or acute respiratory distress syndrome[(1)].

There are three basic radiological patterns of pulmonary infections that we should be able to recognise as well as other 'minor' patterns such as the "ground glass" image whichpresents as a thin, uniformly dense opacity, or the finger-like pattern of allergic bronchopulmonary aspergillosis.

- ALVEOLAR PATTERN. This can be more or less extensive (subsegmental, segmental or lobar), and is the most common radiological expression of pneumonia. It presents as an occupation of the alveolar space, disseminating through the channels of Lambert, and is manifested radiologically as fluffy and homogeneous densities which are ill-defined when not in contact with the pleural surface and usually respects the affected lung volume (Figure 1A). Among variants of the alveolar pattern, or considered by some authors as a fourth independent X-ray pattern[(2)], is the spherical alveolar pattern or round pneumonia which can simulate a lung mass due to its morphology and is more common in children. The alveolar pattern as a mass or not, can occur in conjunction with the bronchogram sign in which the aeration by thin air segments over the area of the consolidation can be seen. With this type of image it is important to include pulmonary hemorrhage, pulmonary edema, disseminated malignancy (usually adenocarcinoma) and, more rarely, alveolar proteinosis (Figure 2) in the differential diagnosis.
- INTERSTITIAL PATTERN. This pattern is recognised by the effect of the pneumonia on pulmonary interstitial inflammation. It manifests as linear, reticular or nodular images often associated with the loss of definition of the bronchovascular contours. An adequate clinical history is needed for the radiological interpretation. Moreover, this pattern may be associated with areas of collapse or subsegmental or placular atelectasia (Figure 1B).
- BRONCHOPNEUMONIA PATTERN. This pattern is the result of the spread of germs through the airway to the pulmonary acinus, and manifests itself as ill-defined nodules on the radiograph. This form of inflammatory lung involvement has a tendency to coalesce towards the inside of the alveolus and therefore may tend towards an alveolar pattern. It can be associated with a component of reduced volume in the affected lung area (Figure 1C).

The different radiological manifestations of pulmonary infections are conditioned by both the host type and his or her immunological levels, as well as by the kind of pathogen involved. A wide range of pathogens may be responsible for pneumonia and the list has continued to grow over recent years. Although the radiographic manifestations are not specific to each type of agent and their identification requires determination by microbiological or indirect serological tests, if we consider the radiological and epidemiological data jointly, we can make a good diagnostic approach to the causal agent. As the majority of cases present with the usual clinical manifestations, this data will be sufficient for us to carry out a successful treatment plan. From an analysis of the overall data we can establish four patient groups: healthy patients, immunocompetent patients with certain diseases or basic predisposing conditions and immunocompromised patients (AIDS vs. non-AIDS).

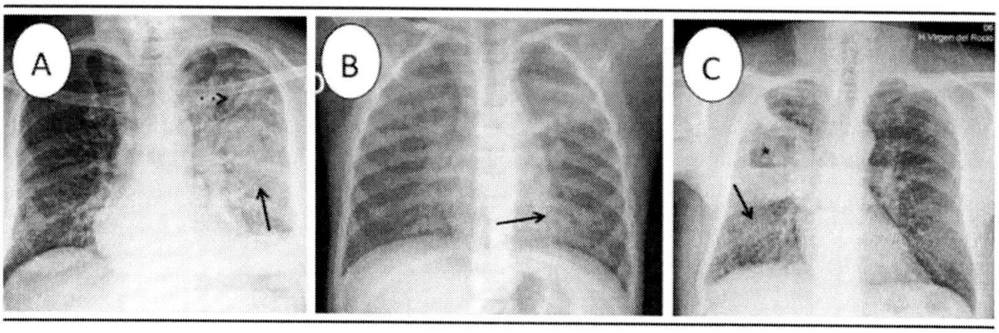

Figure 1. Basic radiological patterns of pneumonia. 1A: Pneumococcal pneumonia manifested as consolidation on the left hemithorax (arrow) with air bronchogram sign (dashed arrow). 1B: linear interstitial pattern in the left lung caused by Epstein-Barr virus (arrow). 1C: bronchopneumonic pattern (arrow) by Pseudomonas aeruginosa in a patient with cavitary lung cancer, note the thick wall cavitary structure, which radiologically means malignant lesion (asterisk).

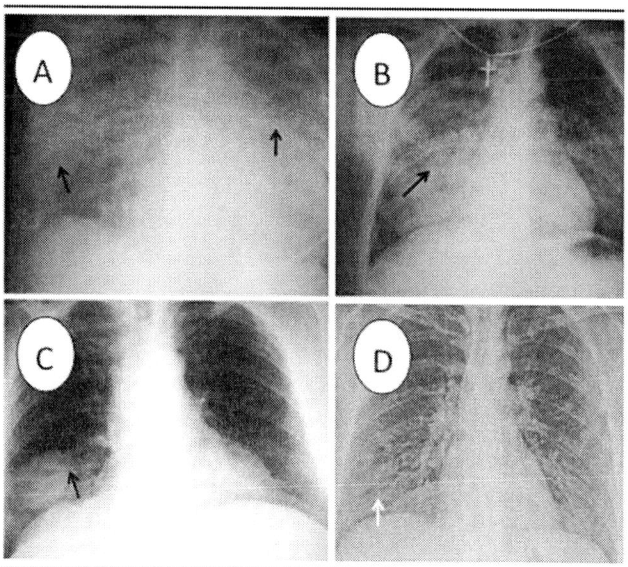

Figure 2. Most common differential diagnosis of alveolar pattern. 2A: cardiogenic pulmonary edema (arrow). Note the increased size of the cardiac silhouette, decompensation cause. 2B: pulmonary hemorrhage (arrow) in a case of Goodpasture syndrome. 2C: Bronchoalveolar carcinoma on middle lobe (arrow). 2D: alveolar proteinosis, which manifests as a 'ground glass' pattern (arrow), which in some cases may mimic inflammatory lung consolidation.

If the patient is healthy the most common diagnostic possibilities are reduced to pneumonia acquired in the community, viral pneumonia and pneumonias caused by atypical pathogens. If the patient is immunocompetent but has an underlying disease or condition (e.g. alcoholism, chronic obstructive pulmonary disease, hospitalization or cancer) we have to add lung infections by aerobic gram-negative germs or other bacteria specific to these risk groups. If the patient is immunocompromised we should give special consideration to fungal infections and certain virus or bacteria that specifically infect this population. In the case of AIDS patients this would mean considering specific etiological agents such as cytomegalovirus, *Pneumocystis jiroveci* or *Aspergillus*, and with non-AIDS patients, agents such as *Candida, Aspergillus* or *Mucor* could be particularly relevant. Therefore it is very important to be familiar with the patient's general health status before considering the imaging diagnostic-etiological possibilities. If the patient is inmucompetent but has compromising health issues or pathologies such as, alcoholism, chronic obstructive pulmonary disease (COPD), hospitalization or neoplasia, we should take into account any agents that can affect both the healthy and immunocompetent group as well as the immunocompetent group under the term 'special'. If the patient is immunocompromised, those agents that may cause pneumonia in both immunocompetent and immunocompromised groups should be included in the differential diagnosis

Obviously not all cases will be completely diagnosed by a single CXR but the integration of imaging and epidemiological findings is a useful tool to establish diagnostic guidelines similar to those already mentioned. The implementation of other complementary studies or even CXRin series (Figure 3) is normally reserved for cases of difficult interpretation, complications or unsatisfactory outcome.

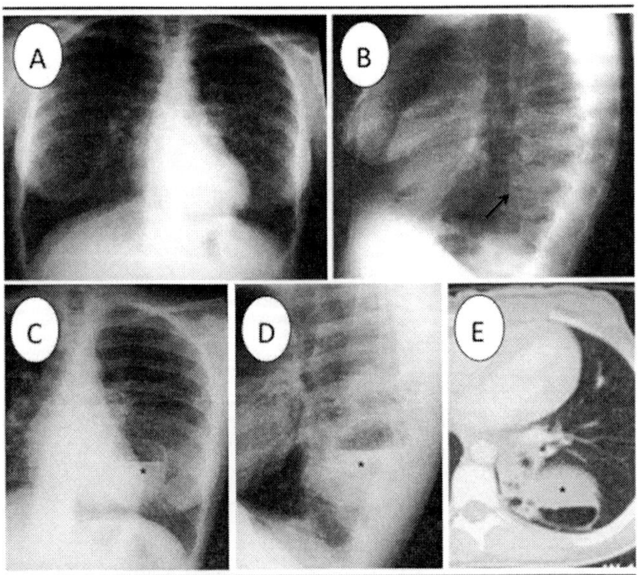

Figure 3. 24 year old male with probable pulmonary sepsis. In a previous study (3A and 3B), a multicystic lesion on posterior left segments was observed(asterisk). This was not easy to recognise on the PA projection, when the patient was asymptomatic. Superinfection of these densities as see fromthe air-fluid level (asterisk) indicated a cystic adenomatoid malformation (MAQ) or sequestration as predisposing factor to infection in the CRX (3C and 3D) and CT with lung parenchyma window(3E). The existence of the MAQ was confirmed during surgery.

Another point worthy of mention isthe chronology of pneumonias. Usually, they are resolved on radiographic follow up within 10-21 days while the few remaining cases might be resolved within about 2 months. A consolidation that lasts more than two months is considered to be a slow resolution and an explanation should be sought for what could be the underlying cause for example, congenital malformation or neoplasm among others(Figure 4) [2].

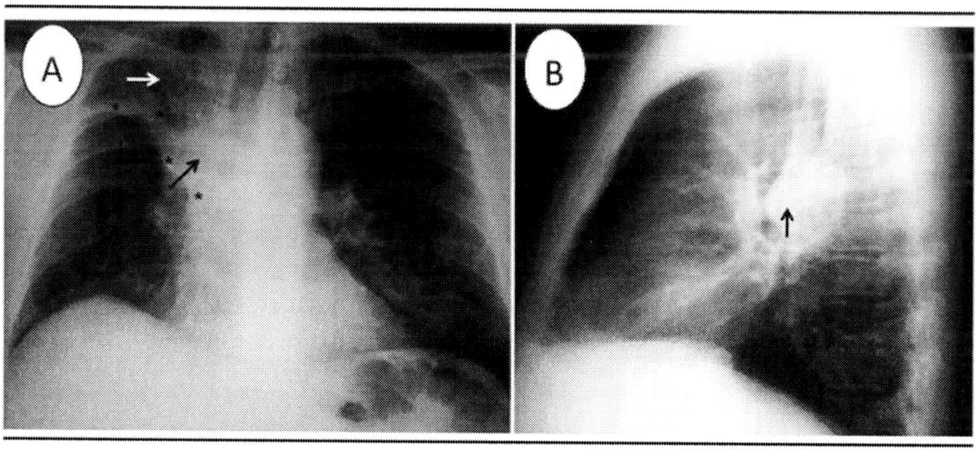

Figure 4. (A: Posteroanterior, B: Lateral). 64 year old male with central lung cancer and postobstructivepneumonitis (with atelectatic component, white arrow) in right upper lobe. Taken together, this sign is known as the 'Golden S' (asterisk), and consists of a concave upward lateral edge, resulting from the collapse, and a concave medial border towards the hilium, resulting from conglomerate mass-central lymph node (black arrow).

1) HEALTHY PATIENTS

We can subdivide this group of patients into three sub-groups:

1. Those in which pneumonia is preceded by pharyngitis, laryngitis and tracheobronchitis symptoms takinginto account the viral etiology,

2. Patients who are part of gated communities (e.g. schools, barracks or prisons) especially if the symptoms could be related to cooling towers or air conditioners, and

3. Healthy individuals, showing a honeycomb pattern on CXR. The members of these three groups fall within the category of community- acquired pneumonia or CAP.

In this last group the CAP is often caused by Gram-positive bacteria, and is a real community health problem as there are between485.000-1.000.000 patients admitted toU.S. hospitals each year for this cause. Up to 90% of community-acquired lobar pneumonia in healthy patients iscaused by two infectious agents:*Streptococcus pneumoniae* (pneumococcus) and *Staphylococcus aureus*. The radiological pattern of this group is usually the alveolar type described above (Figure 5). In detail, it is said that typically,pneumonia from*S. pneumoniae*expands the lung while that caused by *S. Aureus* has a tendency to provoke the formation of cavitation, neumatocele and associated pleural effusion.

Viral pneumonia is the leading cause of respiratory tract infections in the community and usually resolves spontaneously[2]. Clinically, symptoms include runny nose, nasal obstruction, cough and dry throat, and they are often preceded by pharyngitis, laryngitis and tracheobronchitis[1].

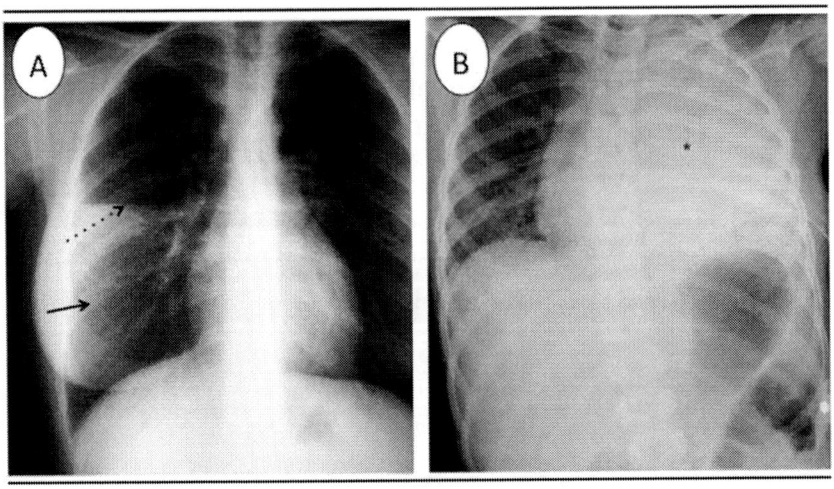

Figure 5. A: 20 year old woman with alveolar pattern in the right lung base with a tendency to coalesce (arrow), suggestive of CAP. From 2-3 days before her visit in the Emergency services, she presented a stuffy nose, cough and dark expectoration, to which 40ºC fever was added on the last day. Pneumococcal antigenuria was positive. Note the well-defined consolidation limits in relation to the cisural surface (dashed arrow) against the poor definition for the rest of the lesion. B: In other cases, pneumococcal pneumonia, can be associated with a major effusion, as seen in this 5 year old girl covering the left hemithorax (asterisk).

In adults, the viruses that commonly cause pneumonia are most often the *Influenza* virus types A and B and *Adenovirus*, not to mention other less prevalent causes such as *chickenpox* virus, *herpes simplex* virus, *Epstein-Barr* or *respiratory syncytial* virus, the latter having a predilection for young children and infants (Figure 6). In the last 25 yearsvery serious viral lung infections have been described, including those caused by*Hantavirus*, *coronavirus* or *influenza* virus of *avian influenza* and the recent H1N1, all of which often have high fever as a common symptom.

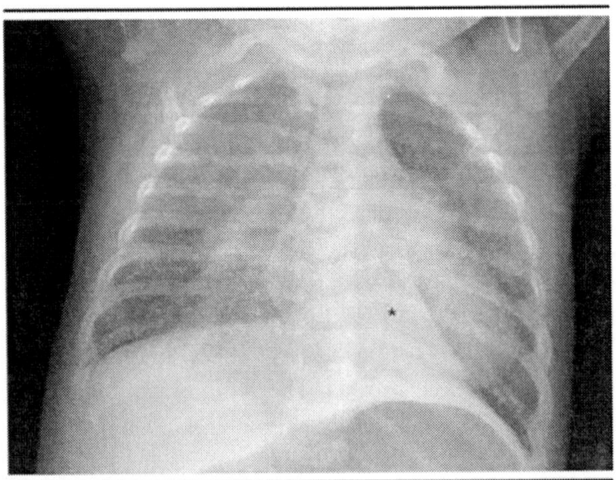

Figure 6. 4 month old baby with basal left lung consolidation (asterisk), corresponding to a RSVlung infection. Note the air bronchogram sign or radiolucency on aerated bronchi, which are distinguished within the radiodensealveolar space occupation. Clinically the baby had breathing difficulty. Symptoms are self-limiting within a few days.

The radiographic findings of viral pneumonia are nonspecific. The predominant pattern is the existence of small, scattered densities which are prone to collect in a mass with a predominantly basal localization and possibly with a 'ground glass pattern' if the *influenza* virus, particularly H1N1, is the causal agent (Figure 7). Some viruses such as *chickenpox* tend to the creation of milimetric size nodular formations(Figure 8) whereas *adenovirus* infections are usually associated with pleural effusion.

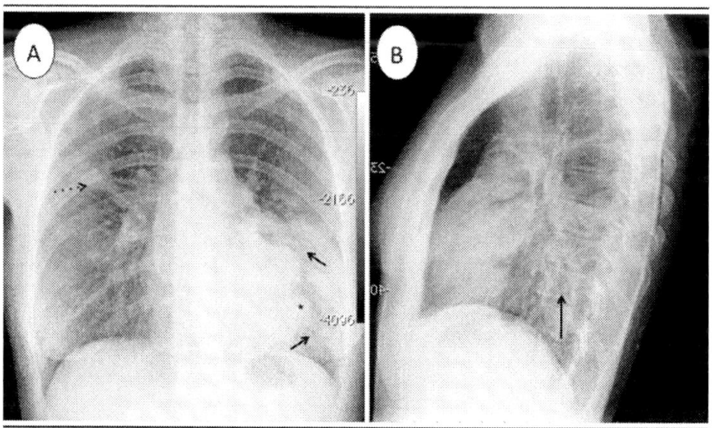

Figure 7. 56 year old woman who complained of fever, left rib pain and malaise of 48 hours duration.Analysis found leukocytosis and increased acute phase reactants. The left paracardial hyperdensity, affecting the whole lung base on that side allows the identification of vascular structures, where a 'ground glass pattern' (arrows) can be seen. A similar picture is visible in the anterior segment of right upper lobe (dashed arrow). The patient also had a thymoma (asterisk). This chest radiography pattern, the presence of flu-like symptoms and multifocality indicates viral pneumonia. Serology confirmed the diagnosis of *Influenza N1H1*.

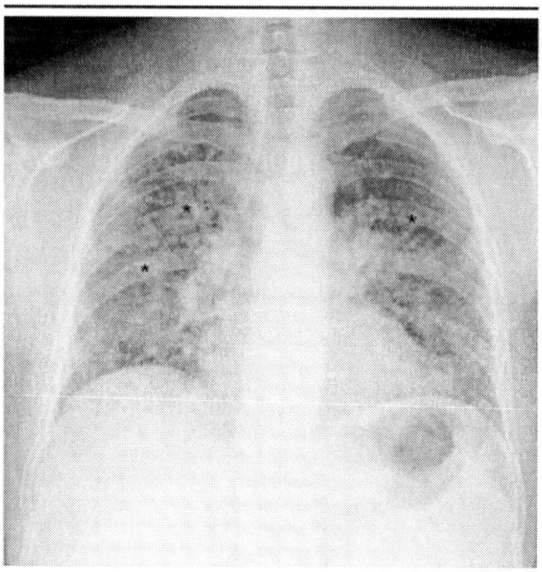

Figure 8. 42 year old male who presented fever, cough, dyspnea, and vesicular rash. A nodular pattern (asterisks) in immunocompetent patients can orient the diagnosis towards atypical or viral pneumonia, as in this case where the responsible germ was the Chickenpox virus.

As previously mentioned, pneumonia can be caused by atypical pathogens including *Mycoplasma pneumoniae*, *Chlamydia pneumoniae* and *Legionella pneumoniae*, For the identification of two of these germs it is often important to recognize the relevance ofthe patient's social context given that *M. pneumoniae* often affects people living in gated communities while the *L. pneumoniae* usually infects people living or working in the vicinity of standing water or closed cooling systems. The typical radiographic pattern of atypical pneumonia is the alveolar or consolidated pattern which has a particularly rapid evolution in the case of *L. Pneomoniae* (Figure 9).

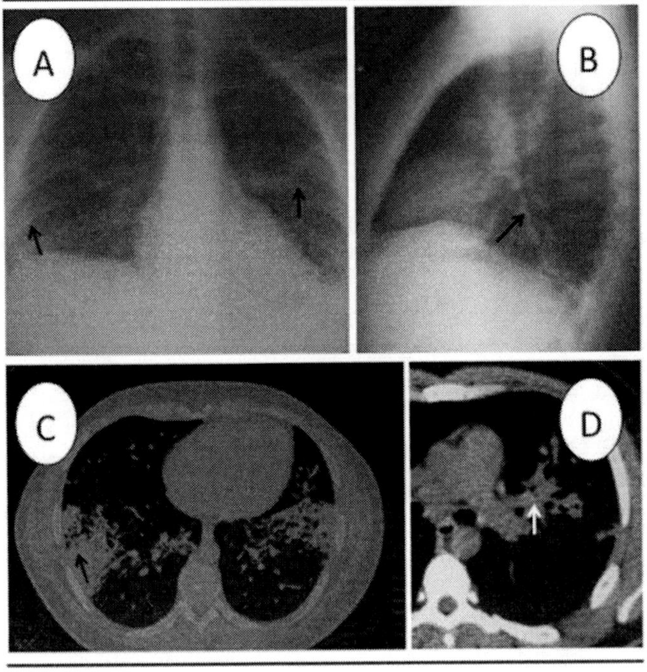

Figure 9. 27 year old male aluminum worker, whose infection begen with fever, dyspnea and nonproductive cough. The patient's occupational history signalled the possibility of atypical pathogens. In this case *Legionella pneumoniae* was isolated. Studies show multiple bilateral alveolar infiltrates (arrow).

2) INMUNOCOMPETENT PATIENTS WITH CERTAIN DISEASES

Although we could make a long list of pneumonia-causing agents associated with certain clinical or sociological contexts or diseases it would not be a very useful classification. Instead, we find that a close examination of the radiological pattern of the pneumonia in question is a more practical way to discover the organism which is responsible for the problem.

Faced with a lobar radiographic pattern, we need to ascertain if the patient has recently suffered a viral or upper respiratory tractinfection and if on the other hand, the radiological pattern is predominantly basal and associated with large pleural effusion or empyema we would be looking at the typical radiological pattern of *Streptococcus pyogenes*. This same radiological pattern, if there is known exposure to *Bacillus anthracis* (e.g. patients in contact with infected goats or goatproducts, especially endemic in parts of Asia) may suggest the diagnosis of anthrax. The clinical setting of pneumonia caused by *Klebsiella pneumoniae* usually includes chronic debilitating diseases like alcoholism andgiven that between 30-50% of *K. Pneumoniae* pneumonias may cavitate,this particular etiology should be consideredwhen cavitation is seen in this risk group This pneumonia is often described as "heavy" due to its association with a large amount of intralveolar inflammatory exudate, which is seen on the radiograph as bulging fissures (Figure 10)[1]. *Haemophilus influenzae*, which is often associated to the existence of malignancy, COPD or alcoholism, usually manifests as multifocal condensation and pleural effusion. *Moraxella catarrhalis*, a typical germ usually causing COPD exacerbation in autumn or early spring, normally presents as a bronchopneumonia with a tendency to coalescence in alveolar densities and pleural effusion. In asthmatic patients, and especially in those with an immediate skin reaction to *Aspergillus fumigatus*, bronchial hypersensitivity to *Aspergillus* may give rise to a special form of fungal pneumonia known as allergic bronchopulmonary aspergillosis.

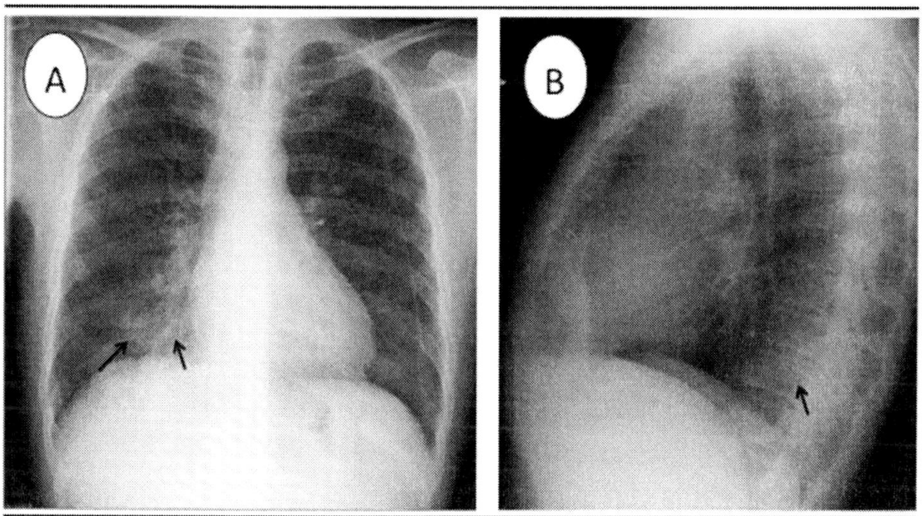

Figure 10. 58 year old male with cardiac transplant, presenting 40°C fever, hypotension and acute renal failure. There is a right basal pulmonary infiltrate (arrows). The rapidly progressive nature of the disease indicated aggressive pneumonia. *K. pneumoniae* bacteremia sensitive to amoxi-clavulanic was obtained and isolated in the peripheral catheter tip.

This condition is characterised by the bronchial filling by hyphae and eosinophilic-rich material that acquires an appearance of 'gloved finger' and manifests itself as finger-like densities predominantly in the upper lobes. In patients with pulmonary cavitation-generating processes (cystic fibrosis, tuberculosis or sarcoidosis), cavitation colonization by *Aspergillus* can lead to intracavitary fungal balls or aspergilloma. In diabetic patients with hematologic malignancies or renal failure, pulmonary mucormycosis is a rare but very aggressive entity. Radiological findings include consolidation areas, nodules and mediastinal and bronchopulmonary lymph nodes which can also be associated with chest wall involvement (Figure 11).

A special situation we have to consider in inmunocompetent individuals is the possibility of hospitalization and so-called nosocomial pneumonia. This is defined as a pneumonia that occurs between 48 and 72 hours after admission and has become the leading cause of hospital death from infection[1]. The microbes that are found most frequently are aerobic Gram-negative (*Pseudomona aeruginosa* or *Enterobacter*),*Staphylococcus*, *H. Influenza* and *S. Pneumoniae*. Viral pneumonias are responsible for a less common group of nosocomial pneumonia. The radiological patterns of each microbe are similar to those described in the various sections of this chapter.

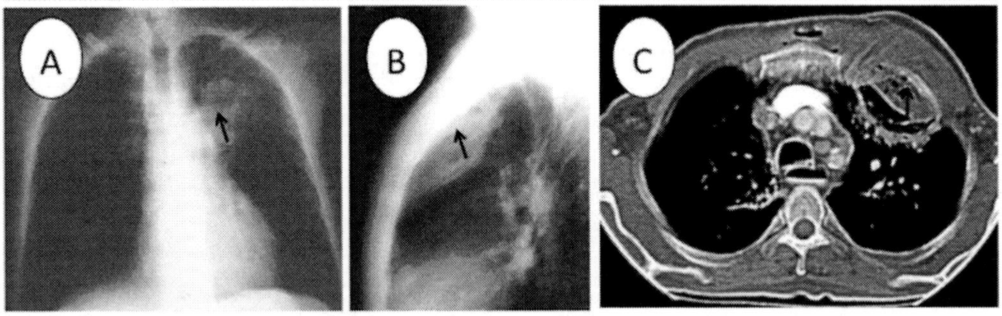

Figure 11. 75 year old male with uncontrolled diabetes, presenting dyspnea, anterior chest wall pain and rusty sputum. The consolidation of the anterior segment of the upper left lobe (arrow) in close contact with the chest wall. The CT confirmed the rib involvement (arrow). *Mucor* was isolated on the biopsy as the germ causing the inflammation.

3) IMMUNOCOMPROMISED NON-AIDS PATIENTS

In addition to the etiological possibilities and the various patterns of pneumonia which can affect immunocompetent individuals, although perhaps with increased virulence and infectivity in the case of immunocompromised patients (Figure 12), this latter group can also be infected by other microbes which are typically grouped into virus and fungi. Pneumonias are the most common cause of consolidation in the immunocompromised host[4].

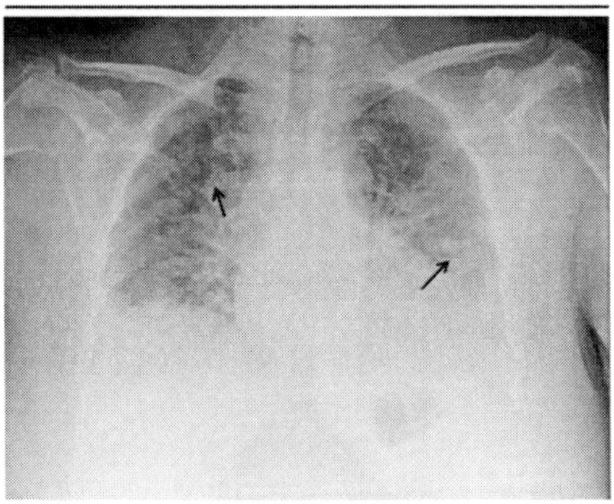

Figure 12. 61 year old woman with a history of IgG lambda multiple myeloma, presenting two days of fever with nonproductive cough and dyspnea with mobilization. The interstitial pattern of both lungs (arrows) in this nosocomial pneumonia raised the possibility of atypical germ vs viral infection, because of the extensive involvement of both lungs. Serology confirmed the existence of *Influenza A*, and the clinical course included a very torpid evolution in the context of her immunosuppression.

Although *Cytomegalovirus* may also affect AIDS patients it can particularly affect non-AIDS immuncompromised patients and is the most common viral infection observed in this group. The risk factors are organ or hematopoietic stem transplantation or prolonged corticosteroid treatment. It usually manifests a ground glass pattern with a tendency to the formation of nodules or to a lesser extent alveolar densities (Figure 13).

Fungal infections such as *Nocardia asteroides* or *Actinomyces israelii* are often observed radiologically as multifocal peripheral densities with a tendency to cavitation that in the case of *N.asteroides* can be associated with a component bronchopneumonic pattern while*A. israelii* is predominantly seen in the lower lobes [3]. Pneumonias caused by *Candida albicans* often exhibit a pattern of bronchopneumonia which on CT scan can be discerned as the presence of millimetric nodules or a pattern of 'tree buds', thus indicating distal airway involvement.

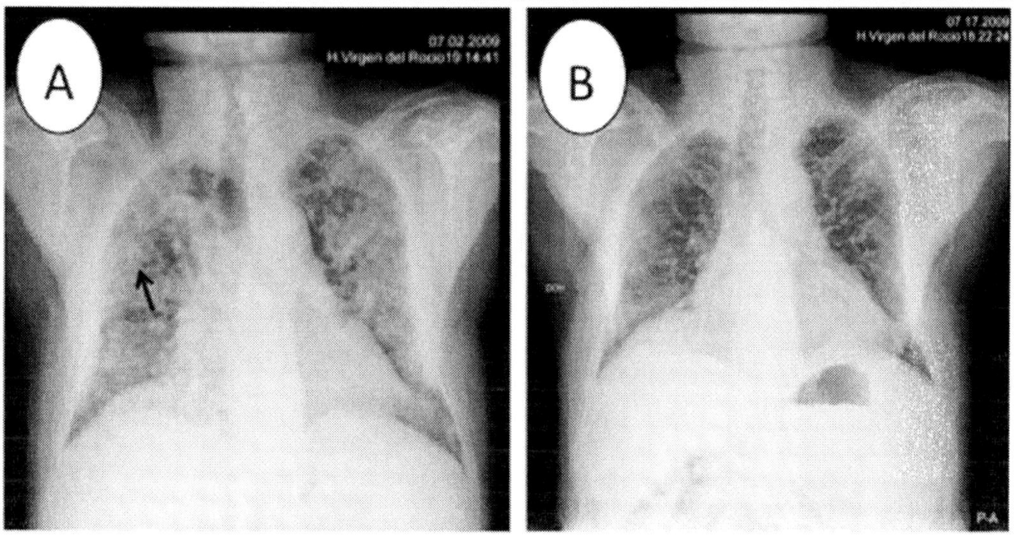

Figure 13.68 year old male with liver transplant, was admitted to ICU for acute renal insufficiency. The clinical symptoms were accompanied with leukocytosis and crackles at auscultation, which started two weeks before admission with irritative dry cough and sore throat with fever up to 39ºC. The history of iatrogenic immunosuppression for trasplant, was a crucial guide to the viral etiology of this case. The pattern of bilateral bronchopneumonia and bilateral nodular lesions (arrows) between the 15 days separating the two figures, gave way to a basic interstitial pattern that was attributed to interstitial lung disease from taking immunosuppressant drugs.

Among the fungal infections *Aspergillus* infection is particularly prevalent. Besides the already mentioned infection possibilities in immunocompetent individuals, superinfection of residual cavities by *Aspergillus* (Figures 14,15), can affect the lungs of immunocompromised patients in three different ways: firstly as angioinvasive in cases of pronounced immunosuppression (Figure 16) which is characterized by nodules surrounded by a halo of ground glass due to perilesional hemorrhage (halo sign) which, when recovery occurs, can acquire an appearance of 'crescent air' or 'semilunar'. Secondly the bronchial invasive form with a pattern of small airway bronchial pneumonia and finally as semi-invasive, in cases of moderate immunosuppression, which manifests as an alveolar pattern with predominant affection of the upper lobe[1,3].

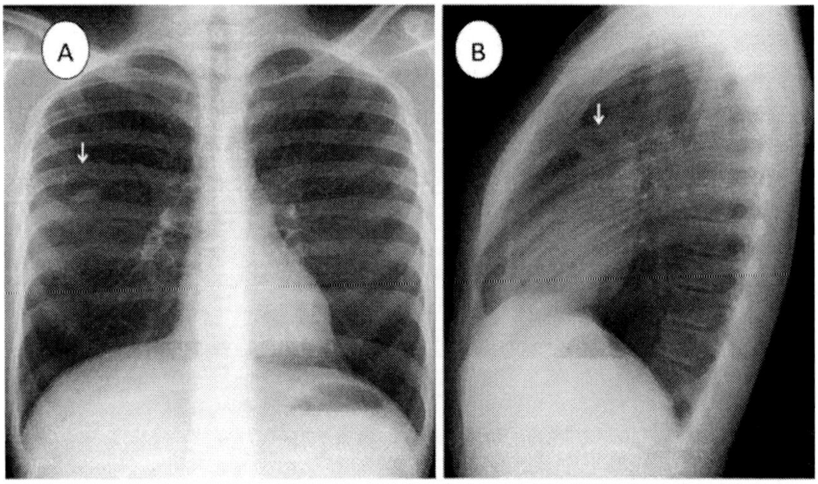

Figure 14. 24 year old male, in treatment for a hematologic malignancy who begins to develop fever. The CXR shows the existence of a cavity with thin and circumscribed borders (arrows, compare with Figure 1C) in the anterior segment of right upper lobe occupied by material in the decline area acquiring the typical appearance of the "intracavitary fungus ball". The patient was treated with antifungals which resolved the occupation image, while cavitation persisted.

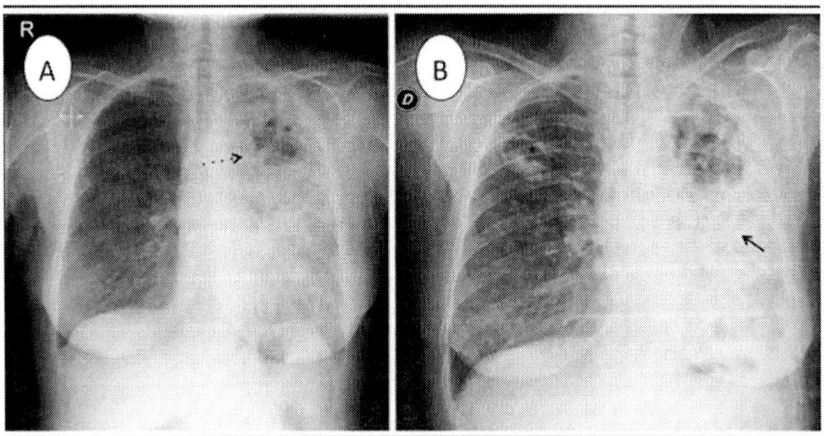

Figure 15. 62 year old women treated with chemotherapy for cervical carcinoma who was admitted with cough and expectoration. The CXR showed a cavitated image in the anterior/apical segment of the upper left lobe (dashed arrow) and alveolar infiltrate in the upper right lobe that cavitated during its evolution (asterisk and arrow). Sputum culture showed Serratia marcensens, and the radiographic pattern was cavitary pneumonia with fungal invasion (aspergilloma) in the lesion of the upper right lobe.

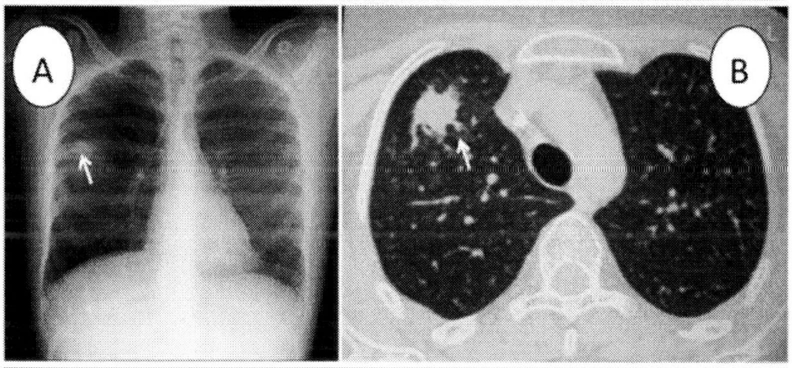

Figure 16. 27 year old male, immunodepressed by bone marrow transplantation presented with fever and respiratory symptoms. The CXR showed an alevolar lesion in the anterior segment of the upper right lobe surrounded by a 'ground glass' halo (arrows) that suggested in this clinical setting the existence of an invasive type of aspergillosis. The peripheral halo corresponds to perilesional hemorrhage due to fungal vascular invasion.

4) IMMUNOCOMPROMISED AIDS PATIENTS

The effect of infectious agents for theimmunosuppressed AIDS patient groupwill vary depending on individual immunosuppression levels (Figure 17). Bacterial infections such as, Rhodococcus (Figures 18, 19) or M. tuberculosis, require a lesser degree of immunocompromise while fungal and Pneumocystis jirovenci infections are more likely to occur with increased immunosuppression, and at even greater levels lung infections by Mycobacterium avium intracellular and *Cytomegalovirus* will appear.

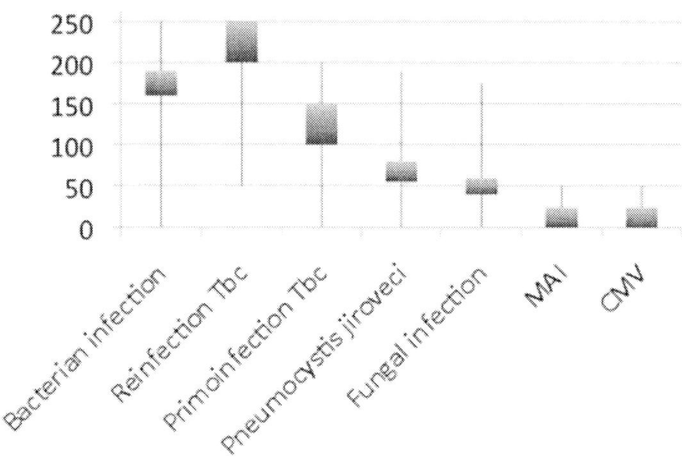

Figure 17.The pulmonary infections spectrum in AIDS patients. The coordinate axis represents the number of CD4 + / UL. The line represents the range where the infection may be and the drawer the levels where it is most common. Adapted from Reference 1.

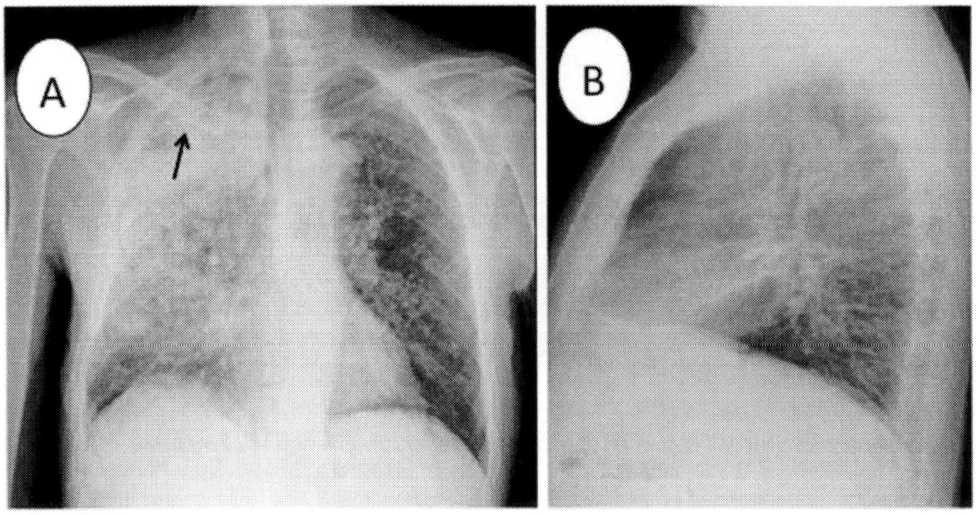

Figure 18. 43 year old male, HIV positive CD4 + 58c/UL and granulomatous tuberculosis sequel, who presented clinical symptoms of cough with mucopurulent expectoration, and occasionally hemoptysis of 7 days duration, an alveolar occupation (arrow) with discrete right lung volume expansion related to bacterial CAP.

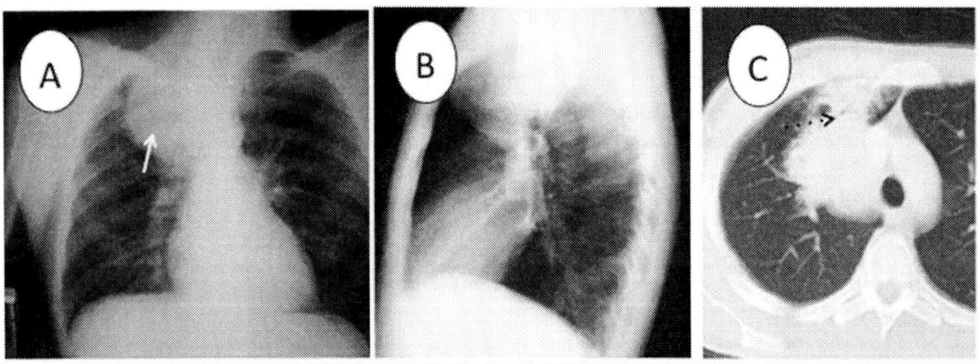

Figure 19. 47 year old male, HIV positive, with fever and pneumonia symptoms. On the conventional chest study a lung mass was discovered (arrow). The CT showed air bronchogram within the lesion (dashed arrow). The final diagnosis was a *Rodoccocus* motivated abscess.

P. jirovenci involvementmay manifest as a diffuse symmetrical perihilar alveolar pattern which may progress within a few days to affect the entire lung with focal areas of ground glass and the possible appearance of microcysts from bronchiolar damage. However, in up to 10-39% of cases the CXR may be normal[(3,4)] (Figure 20). This microorganism produces pneumonia in 60% of patients with AIDS and is responsible for more than a third of the deaths in this population[(5)]. The other fungal infections (cryptococcal, histoplasmosis, blastomycosis, or coccidioidomycosis) usually present with a diffuse micronodular (miliary)interstitial pattern type.

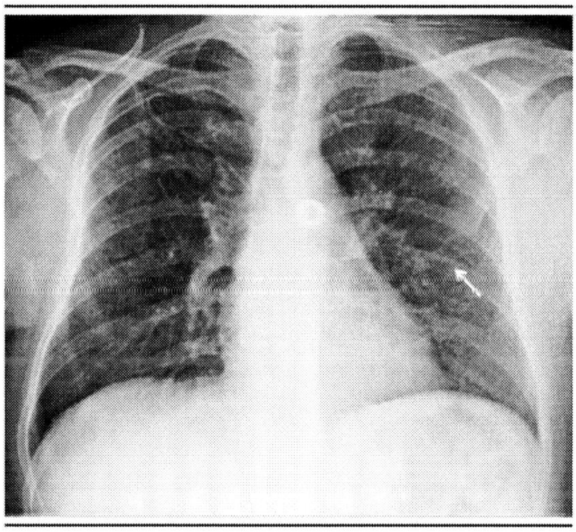

Figure 20. 45 year old male HIV positive and Hodgkin's lymphoma in chemotherapy treatment. Initial torpid evolution with development of acute respiratory failure and focusing of respiratory symptoms (nonproductive cough.) The ground glass pattern (arrow) in this clinical context guided the radiological management. After initiation of empiric treatment for *Pneumocystis* with cotrimoxazole and steroids, the patient began to evolve favorably with marked improvement. On leaving hospital he was eupneic, afebrile and asymptomatic.

A discussion of tuberculosis (TB) pneumonia with regard to this group is necessary because, although it may occur in immuncompetent individuals, its incidence is up to 200-500 times higher in HIV-positive patients[(1)]. It is estimated that 25% of seropositive patients have active TB. Its radiographic pattern consists of an alveolar type affecting predominantly upper and posterior lung segments in cases of primary affectation and a bronchogenic spread pattern or bronchopneumonic pattern in cases of re-infection (Figure 21). In about 30-60% of patients the presence of lymphadenopathy can be seen seen on CXR[(1)]. Finally, it should be remembered that low immunedepression is not a necessary condition for the revival of previous TB in AIDS patients, unlike the case of primary tuberculous infection that does require a heightened state of immunosuppression.

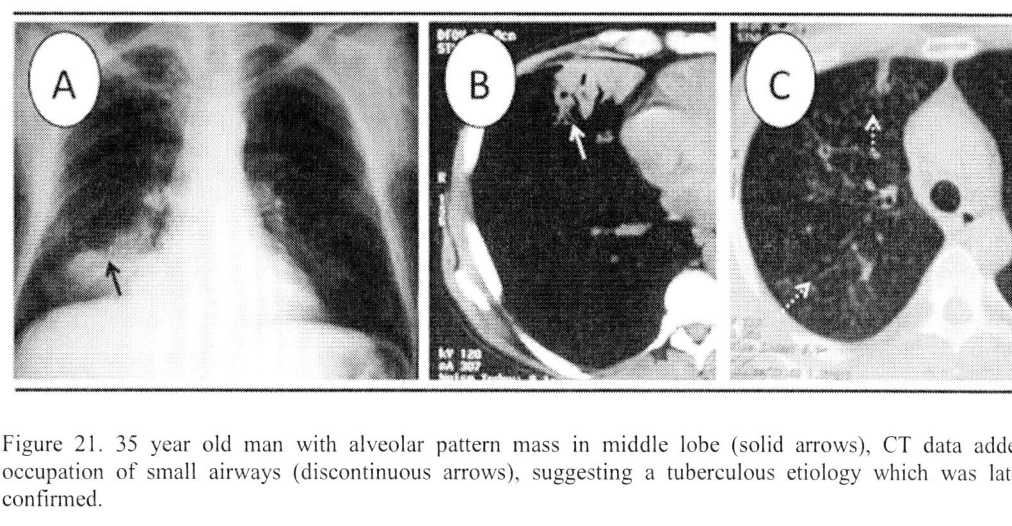

Figure 21. 35 year old man with alveolar pattern mass in middle lobe (solid arrows), CT data added occupation of small airways (discontinuous arrows), suggesting a tuberculous etiology which was later confirmed.

To conclude we can affirm that once we have analyzed the clinical context and understood its implications, the observed radiological patterns will be of vital importance in the diagnosis of each case, something which is fundamental for the correct management and treatment of these patients.

Bibliography

[1] Franquet T. Infecciones pulmonares. *En: Radiología Esencial*. Ed. Panamericana. Ed Del Cura JL, Pedraza S, Gayete A. Madrid, 2.010. Pp: 156-176.

[2] Hansell, Armstrong, Lynch y McAdams. Infecciones de los pulmones y la pleura. *En Tórax. Diagnóstico radiológico*. 4ta Edición. Ed Marbán. Oxford, 2.008. Pp: 163-244.

[3] Gotway M, Berger W, Leung J. Infecciones pulmonares. *En Radiología Pulmonar y Cardiovascular*. Ed Marbán, Webb y Higgins. Philadelphia, 2.009. Pp: 357-405.

[4] Moreno MD, Alcántara R. Complicaciones pulmonares en el SIDA y en el paciente inmunocomprometido no-SIDA. *En: Diagnóstico por Imagen del tórax: Tomografía Computerizada y Resonancia Magnética*. Ed. Caduce. Sevilla, 2.006. Pp: 319-343.

[5] Hoover DR, Saah AJ, Barcellar H, et al. Clinical manifestactions of AIDS in the era of Pneumocystis profilaxis. *N Engl J med* 1993; 329: 1922-6.

Index

D

N

O

P

Q

R

S

T

U

V